The Omega-Factor

Omega-3 fatty acids can limit the inflammation that is the underlying cause of many severe diseases of modern civilization, including diabetes and cardiovascular disease. *The Omega-Factor: Promoting Health, Preventing Premature Aging and Reducing the Risk of Sudden Cardiac Death* presents information on the mechanisms whereby inflammation damages organs and the blood vessels serving them, as well as the hard science on the mechanisms by which the omega-3 fatty acids protect those tissues. It also features peer-reviewed evidence from clinical trials on these topics.

The book gives cutting-edge information from state-of-the-art developments such as the test that can be done to measure the omega-3 status of one's own tissues, the "Omega-3 Index," which can give many years of early warning so that one can take preventive steps and decrease the odds of a heart attack, stroke or kidney disease. It explains why a Mediterranean Diet plan rich in omega-3 and omega-6 fatty acids is protective, and it features a six-day meal plan with recipes that will improve body levels of omega-3s. This book helps readers understand the differences between various sources of omega-3 fatty acids, namely flaxseed vs fish oil vs algae-derived oils.

Features

- Provides evidence-based information on why blood vessels require omega-3 fatty acids to maintain health
- Details best sources of the various fatty acids, including plant-based sources.
- Includes "at-home tests" to assess cardiovascular status
- Presents literature on how to improve chances of avoiding heart attacks, peripheral arterial disease, strokes, kidney disease and Type 2 diabetes

The Omega-Factor: Promoting Health, Preventing Premature Aging and Reducing the Risk of Sudden Cardiac Death is an essential resource for healthcare professionals, clinicians and dietitians, as well as for the reader who aims to achieve the goal of a much longer health-span, not just a longer lifespan.

Robert Fried, PhD, is a cardiovascular physiologist and NY State Licensed Clinical Psychologist. He is Emeritus Professor, doctoral faculty in Behavioral Neurosciences, City University of New York (CUNY). He has published more than a dozen academic and trade books on cardiovascular health, nutrition and human sexuality, and more than 50 peer-reviewed scientific journal publications. Fried holds several US patents in biomedical instrumentation and he is listed in the year 2000 (Century) Marquis's Who's Who.

Richard M. Carlton, MD, is an integrative physician who includes complementary and alternative approaches in the treatment of numerous medical problems, including migraines, inflammatory bowel disease and diabetes. He is formerly Principal Staff Physician, Rehabilitation Research Institute (RRI), ICD-International Center for the Disabled, New York, NY.

The Omega-Factor

Promoting Health, Preventing Premature Aging and Reducing the Risk of Sudden Cardiac Death

Robert Fried, PhD
Richard M. Carlton, MD

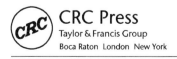

CRC Press is an imprint of the
Taylor & Francis Group, an **informa** business

First edition published 2023
by CRC Press
6000 Broken Sound Parkway NW, Suite 300, Boca Raton, FL 33487-2742

and by CRC Press
4 Park Square, Milton Park, Abingdon, Oxon, OX14 4RN
CRC Press is an imprint of Taylor & Francis Group, LLC

© 2023 Taylor & Francis Group, LLC

Reasonable efforts have been made to publish reliable data and information, but the author and publisher cannot assume responsibility for the validity of all materials or the consequences of their use. The authors and publishers have attempted to trace the copyright holders of all material reproduced in this publication and apologize to copyright holders if permission to publish in this form has not been obtained. If any copyright material has not been acknowledged please write and let us know so we may rectify in any future reprint.

Except as permitted under U.S. Copyright Law, no part of this book may be reprinted, reproduced, transmitted, or utilized in any form by any electronic, mechanical, or other means, now known or hereafter invented, including photocopying, microfilming, and recording, or in any information storage or retrieval system, without written permission from the publishers.

For permission to photocopy or use material electronically from this work, access www.copyright.com or contact the Copyright Clearance Center, Inc. (CCC), 222 Rosewood Drive, Danvers, MA 01923, 978-750-8400. For works that are not available on CCC please contact mpkbookspermissions@tandf.co.uk

Trademark notice: Product or corporate names may be trademarks or registered trademarks and are used only for identification and explanation without intent to infringe.

ISBN: 978-1-032-45098-8 (hbk)
ISBN: 978-1-032-40941-2 (pbk)
ISBN: 978-1-003-35546-5 (ebk)

DOI: 10.1201/b23284

Typeset in Times
by Deanta Global Publishing Services, Chennai, India

Contents

Foreword xi
Preface xv
Disclaimer xvii
Acknowledgments xix

Chapter 1   What Is the Omega-Factor? 1

    1.1   The Myth of the Paleolithic Gourmet 1
    1.2   Omega-3 Fatty Acids Save Lives 2
    1.3   Fats—A Primer 4
    1.4   What Is Cholesterol? 6
    1.5   What Are "Triglycerides?" 6
    1.6   The Omega-6/Omega-3 Ratio 7
    1.7   The Omega-3 Index (O3I) 8
    1.8   Omega-6 and Omega-3 Fatty Acids 9
        1.8.1   Omega-3s, of a Type, Save Lives 11
    1.9   Omega-6 Fatty Acids 11
    1.10   How Meaningful Is the Omega-6 to Omega-3 Ratio? 12
    1.11   How to Find Out Our Omega-3 Index (O3I) 13
    1.12   The Importance of the Omega-3 Index (O3I) 14
    1.13   Your *Hot-Rod* Mitochondria 16
    1.14   There's No Free Lunch 16
    1.15   The *Three Fates* 17
    References 19

Chapter 2   If You Ate What They Ate in Okinawa 23

    2.1   Introduction 23
    2.2   Omega-3s Are Principally Powerfully "Antioxidants:"
        Why Do We Need Antioxidants? 23
    2.3   We Hate Them But We Can't Do without Them 24
    2.4   They Live Longer in Okinawa Because They Don't Eat
        What You Eat 25
        Why do Okinawans live longer on average than we do? 27
    2.5   Antioxidants—The Quicker Picker-Upper 27
    2.6   The Antioxidants the Body Makes 28
        Exogenous antioxidants include 28
        2.6.1   The Antioxidant Paradox 29
    2.7   Resveratrol for What Ails You 29
    2.8   What Is ORAC? How Much Do We Need? 30
    2.9   No Good Deed Goes Unpunished 31

		2.10 It Takes 2 Pounds of Blueberries to Get the ORAC of 100 Grams of Flaxseed 33

Chapter 3 Omegas Strengthen Your Blood Vessels and Your Heart 39

- 2.10.1 Caveat 36
- References 36

Chapter 3 Omegas Strengthen Your Blood Vessels and Your Heart 39

- 3.1 What You Don't Know Surely Will Hurt You 39
- 3.2 It's a Gas 41
- 3.3 How a Simple "Blunder" Explains Cardiovascular and Heart Disease 42
- 3.4 How Does Diet Damage the Endothelium? 43
- 3.5 Healthy Food Patterns vs Unhealthy Food Patterns 44
  - 3.5.1 High-Sodium Diet 44
  - 3.5.2 High-Animal Fat Diet 44
  - 3.5.3 High-Carbohydrate Diet 45
- 3.6 At the Heart of the Matter 46
- 3.7 Arterial Vessel Compliance 49
- 3.8 Flaxseed Oil Promotes Arterial Blood Vessel Elasticity (Compliance) 50
- 3.9 Omega-3s "Lubricate" Your Heart Valves 51
- 3.10 Omega-3s Protect the Coronary Arteries 52
- 3.11 Omega-3 Fatty Acids and Cardiovascular Disease: New Recommendations from the American Heart Association (2003) 54
- References 56

Chapter 4 Omega-3s and Hypertension, Atherosclerosis and Type 2 Diabetes 59

- 4.1 Essential Hypertension 59
- 4.2 What Are the Dangers of High Blood Pressure? 60
- 4.3 We Are What We Didn't Eat 62
- 4.4 Blood Pressure and the Omega-3 Index (O3I) 64
- 4.5 Omega-3 Fatty Acids Reduce the Inflammation Process in Atherosclerosis 66
- 4.6 Omega-3s May Prevent Atherosclerosis and Stabilize, Even Reduce, Plaque 67
- 4.7 Omega-3 Fatty Acids Can Reduce Coronary Artery Plaque 68
- 4.8 Lignans in Flaxseed Slow Progression of Atherosclerosis 68
- 4.9 Type 2 Diabetes—Ants Know It Long Before You Do 69
- 4.10 Long-Term Intake of Omega-3 Fatty Acids from Fish Lowers the Risk of Developing Type 2 Diabetes 70
- 4.11 Omega-3 Fatty Acids and Heart and Blood Vessel Disease in Type 2 Diabetes 71
- 4.12 Omega-3 Fatty Acids and Peripheral Neuropathy 71

Contents

	4.13	Omega-3 Fatty Acids Benefits in Type 2 Diabetes Eye Damage (Retinopathy)—The Secret Revealed 72
	4.14	Omega-3 Fatty Acids Improve Diabetic Slow Wound-Healing 73
	References 73

Chapter 5 Peripheral Artery Disease, Arthritis, Chronic Kidney Disease, Irritable Bowel Syndrome, Glaucoma, Age-Related Macular Degeneration and Mild Cognitive Impairment in Aging 77

    5.1   Where's the Fire? 77
    5.2   Peripheral Artery Disease and Claudication 79
    5.3   The Ankle-Brachial Index (ABI) 79
    5.4   The ABI and Endothelial Dysfunction 82
    5.5   Omega-3 Fatty Acid Deficiency in Peripheral Artery Disease 82
           5.5.1   The Higher Body Omega-3 Fatty Acids, the Higher the ABI 82
    5.6   Osteo- and Rheumatoid Arthritis 83
    5.7   Omega-3 Fatty Acids Improve Filtration in Chronic Kidney Disease 84
           5.7.1   Omega-3s from Fish Oil Improve Quality of Life in Dialysis Patients 86
    5.8   Irritable Bowel Syndrome (IBS) 86
    5.9   Glaucoma and Macular Degeneration 87
           5.9.1   A Paradox 88
    5.10   Omega-3 Fatty Acid DHA Protects Vision 90
    5.11   Brain Fish Oil-Lube for Mild Cognitive Impairment in Aging 90
           5.11.1 Inflamm-aging 90
    References 92

Chapter 6 Flax I: A Pharaoh's Garment, a Roman's Laxative 99

    6.1   Those Blue Flower Roadside Weeds? 99
    6.2   Flax Is a "Functional Food" 100
    6.3   Cyanogenic Glycosides (CNGs) 102
    6.4   Disclaimer 104
    6.5   Caveat 105
    6.6   (Almost) Everything You'd Want to Know about Flaxseed 105
           6.6.1   Supplement Dosages in Published Clinical Trials 107
    6.7   Chronic Systemic Inflammation 109
    6.8   Inflammation in Metabolic Syndrome (Read Endothelial Dysfunction) 109
           6.8.1   Metabolic Syndrome 109
    6.9   Inflammation in Ulcerative Colitis 110

	6.10	Cardiovascular Risk Factors	110
	6.11	Coronary Artery Disease	110
	6.12	Abnormal Serum Lipids	110
	6.13	Cardiovascular Risk Factors	110
	6.14	Type 2 Diabetes	110
		6.14.1 Type 2 Diabetes with Mild Hypercholesterolemia	111
	6.15	Lupus Nephritis	111
	6.16	Obesity and Insulin Resistance	111
	6.17	Systemic Inflammation in Morbid Obesity	111
	6.18	Prostate Cancer	111
	6.19	Rheumatoid Arthritis	111
	6.20	Osteoarthritis—Flaxseed Poultice Compress	111
	6.21	Chronic Kidney Disease	112
	6.22	Chronic Kidney Disease: Inflammation and Oxidative Stress in Hemodialysis	112
	6.23	Polycystic Ovary Syndrome	112
		6.23.1 Hormonal Levels in Polycystic Ovarian Syndrome	112
	References		112
Chapter 7	Flax Is Good for You—At-Home Supplementation		117
	7.1	But, What's Good for the Goose …	117
	7.2	Published Supplementation Recommendations	117
	7.3	Supplementation vs Adjunct Treatment	119
	7.4	Tracking Omega-3 Fatty Acid Intake: The Omega-3 Index	121
	7.5	Organic vs Non-Organic Flaxseeds?	122
	7.6	Golden Flaxseed vs Brown Flaxseed	123
	7.7	Whole Flaxseed vs Ground Flaxseed or Flax Meal	123
	7.8	Flax Oil	125
	7.9	Including Flaxseed in Daily Diet	125
	7.10	Flaxseed Recipe Books	127
	7.11	Caveat	127
	Note		128
	References		128
Chapter 8	Flax Is Good: Fish and Other Sea Critters Are Better		131
	8.1	Phytoplankton 101	131
		8.1.1 Caveat	133
	8.2	But Before We Get to Fish …	133
	8.3	The Mediterranean Diet Score (MDS) vs the Omega-6:3 Ratio	135
	8.4	What Is a Fish?	135
		8.4.1 Tilapia: Benefits and Cautions	139
	8.5	Health Benefits of Fish	139

8.6	Cooking Fish	139
8.7	Fish—Home Delivery	140
8.8	Fish May Have Contaminants and Dangerously High Levels of Mercury	140
	8.8.1 Concerning Mercury	141
8.9	Shellfish Are Not Fish	142
8.10	Fish Oil	143
	8.10.1 A Note on Cod Liver Oil	144
8.11	Eels	145
8.12	Fish Roe/Caviar, Sea Urchin and Seaweed	146
8.13	Shrimp, Prawn and Lobster	147
	8.13.1 Krill and Krill Oil	148
8.14	Shellfish Allergy Is Not Likely to Be Iodine Allergy	148
8.15	Octopus and Squid	150
	8.15.1 Caveat	150
8.16	Oysters and Clams	151
8.17	Scallops	151
8.18	Covid-19—Shellfish to the Rescue	152
8.19	Jellyfish	155
8.20	Mussels and Abalone	155
8.21	Caveat	156
References		156

Chapter 9 Omega-3 Target and Six-Day Meals Plan 159

9.1	Before You Head for the Kitchen	159
9.2	Omega-3 Index Target: 8.0%	159
9.3	Some Plant Sources of Omega-3 Fatty Acids	160
9.4	How to Determine the Omega-3 Fatty Acid Composition of Meals	162
	9.4.1 Some Sources of Omega-3-Rich Recipes	162
9.5	Breakfast Recipes	162
	9.5.1 Hearty Oatmeal Pancakes with Flax and Chia Seeds	162
	9.5.2 Blueberry Omega-3 Breakfast Bowl	163
	9.5.3 Homemade Açaí Bowl	164
	9.5.4 Mini Blueberry Muffin Recipe	164
	9.5.5 Greek Muffin-Tin Omelets with Feta and Peppers	165
	9.5.6 Mediterranean Tofu Scramble	166
9.6	Lunch Recipes	167
	9.6.1 Mediterranean Shrimp Quinoa Bowl Recipe	167
	9.6.2 Mexican Sardine Salad Stuffed Avocados	167
	9.6.3 Salmon Cakes with Creamy Ginger-Sesame Sauce	168
	9.6.4 Tuna and Green Bean Salad	169

		9.6.5	Spinach Salad with Winter Squash and Walnuts 170
		9.6.6	Grilled Sauerkraut Avocado Sandwich 170
	9.7	Dinner Recipes 171
		9.7.1	Green Tea Poached Salmon with Ginger Lime Sauce 171
		9.7.2	Baked Mediterranean Fish Recipe 172
		9.7.3	Simply Poached Salmon.. 173
		9.7.4	Salmon Salad with Parsley and Capers.................... 173
		9.7.5	Slow-Roasted Salmon with Fennel, Citrus and Chiles... 174
		9.7.6	Harvest Squash Medley... 174
	9.8	Optional Desserts 175
References 175
Index.. 177

Foreword

The relationship between marine-derived omega-3 polyunsaturated fatty acids (PUFAs) and cardiovascular disease (CVD) originated from the landmark research conducted by Bang and Dyerberg in 1971. They reported a low incidence of ischemic heart disease in Greenland's Inuit population, an isolated cohort with a diet composed primarily of whales, seals, sea birds and fish. Compared to a Danish cohort, the Inuit had a less atherogenic blood lipid profile, higher omega-3 polyunsaturated fatty acids (PUFAs) in platelet membranes and longer blood clotting times. Bang and Dyerberg postulated that the low incidence of CVD was a consequence of the distinct dietary pattern high in the marine-derived omega-3 PUFAs, eicosapentaenoic acid (EPA) and docosahexaenoic acid (DHA).

These seminal findings created a new nutrition research frontier about how omega-3 PUFAs affect CVD and other chronic diseases, as well as overall health. The benefits are illustrated by a recent pooled analysis of 17 international epidemiologic studies (with 42,466 individuals that were followed for an average of 16 years). It was found that the risk for death from all causes was significantly lower (by 15–18%) in the highest versus the lowest quintile of circulating omega-3 fatty acids (EPA, DHA and another omega-3 fatty acid, docosapentaenoic acid). Similar benefits were seen for death from CVD, cancer and other causes.

In terms of fish/seafood consumption, studies have demonstrated that two to three servings of fish per week are associated with a lower incidence of all-cause mortality, CVD, coronary heart disease, myocardial infarction, stroke and heart failure. Collectively, over the past 50+ years, we have learned much about the effects of omega-3 fatty acids on the metabolic processes that underlie the development and progression of leading chronic diseases. We have also developed an extensive understanding of the biological mechanisms that account for the impressive health benefits of omega-3 fatty acids.

Chronic diseases are the leading cause of morbidity and mortality, both in the United States and globally. Poor diet and high blood pressure are the two top modifiable risk factors for chronic diseases. Overall, diet quality in the United States is poor with an average Healthy Eating Index score (a measure of diet quality) that is less than 60% of ideal. Intake of vegetables, fruits, whole grains, dairy products and seafood are woefully under-consumed, with only 10% of the U.S. population meeting dietary recommendations for seafood (i.e., at least two servings of fatty fish per week). In addition, Americans over-consume saturated fat, sodium and added sugars. Estimates of omega-3 fatty acid intake in the United States are as low as 100 mg/day, which fall far short of the 250 mg/day that is recommended. Given that seafood is the major dietary source of omega-3 fatty acids, it is clear that seafood consumption must increase. Consumption of 8 ounces of seafood per week provides approximately 250 mg EPA + DHA per day.

Based on the preponderance of evidence, the American Heart Association in its 2021 Scientific Statement, Dietary Guidance to Improve Cardiovascular Health, recommends healthy sources of protein (of which fish/seafood is a healthy protein source) and specifically recommends at least two fish meals per week as part of a healthy dietary pattern. The greatest benefits occur when seafood replaces foods high in saturated fatty acids (SFAs). Global seafood recommendations are similar to this guidance—the average seafood recommendation is one to two servings per week in European countries. Beyond authoritative recommendations for seafood consumption, the Food and Drug Administration has issued a Qualified Health Claim for omega-3 fatty acids: "Supportive but not conclusive research shows that consumption of EPA and DHA omega-3 fatty acids may reduce the risk of coronary heart disease."

Science has convincingly shown how healthy omega-3 fatty acids can make us. Now, the quest is to get the word out to the public to encourage increased consumption of seafood omega-3 fatty acids to benefit health. This book, *The Omega Factor*, by Drs. Robert Fried and Richard Carlton is a noble effort that communicates the many virtues of omega-3 fatty acids.

In Chapter 1, there is a very good overview on fats and fatty acids and their metabolism. Different types of fats and the major individual fatty acids in our diets are discussed. Important food sources of these different fats and fatty acids are described. This chapter is where readers will learn about the Omega-3 Index, which is a valuable tool that can be used for monitoring whether omega-3 fatty acid intake is adequate. Useful information is presented about how to check your Omega-3 Index. In Chapter 2, the significance of having a good antioxidant status is emphasized—this is important to prevent oxidative stress and the health problems associated with it. Both a healthy diet and omega-3 fatty acids are potent antioxidants, protecting against many chronic diseases that are caused by oxidative stress. Chapter 3 provides a very good overview about the health benefits of omega-3 fatty acids on the circulatory system and the heart. A healthy vascular system is dependent on a healthy diet (including omega-3 fatty acids), which promotes nitric oxide production and blood vessel elasticity. In contrast, a poor diet damages the blood vessel endothelium, hinders nitric oxide production and causes arterial stiffness (rigidity), thereby adversely affecting blood flow. The beneficial effects of omega-3 fatty acids on the endothelium (and the constituent endothelial cells that line all blood vessels) are also discussed in Chapter 5. The focus of Chapter 4 is on the role of omega-3 fatty acids in reducing inflammation and decreasing risk of plaque rupture. A ruptured plaque activates the clotting cascade, increasing the risk of a heart attack or a stroke. Omega-3 fatty acids stabilize plaques and lower the risk of plaque rupture and heart attack, stroke and cardiac death/sudden cardiac death. Low-grade chronic inflammation is linked to many other chronic diseases such as diabetes, chronic kidney disease, cognitive impairment and age-related eye diseases (such as glaucoma and macular degeneration). The research showing protective associations between omega-3 fatty acids and some of these diseases may be due to their anti-inflammatory properties. Chapters 6 and 7 overview the benefits of plant-based omega-3 fatty acids (primarily alpha-linolenic acid) for health. Readers can access many delicious flax recipes. In Chapter 8, the type and amount of omega-3 fatty acids from flax and many types of seafood are compared—this is where information can be found about how much omega-3 fatty acids are present in different seafood species. This chapter also includes recipes that can be accessed for different types of seafood. In Chapter 9, many valuable resources are listed and there is also a six-day meal plan with recipes included that provides a good starting point for planning a healthy diet. The reader will benefit from the many interesting tables and figures that nicely complement the text and, also, serve as a good resource.

A key takeaway from the book is that it is important to consume adequate amounts of omega-3 fatty acids (principally from fish/seafood but also other sources) for good health. Critically important to this is knowing your Omega-3 Index to assure that you are consuming sufficient quantities of these essential fatty acids that are central to achieving and maintaining good health. Be sure to monitor your Omega-3 Index on a routine basis to guarantee you are getting the maximum benefits of these wonderful fatty acids for your health.

In summary, the book reinforces the importance of including seafood in a healthy diet and why omega-3 fatty acids are so good for you. To your health!

Penny M. Kris-Etherton, PhD, RD
Evan Pugh University Professor of Nutritional Sciences
Department of Nutritional Sciences
Penn State University
University Park, Pennsylvania

Preface

It has been our practice to convert the references in the full-length journal articles from sundry journal or any other styles to a more or less AMA style to help you to follow up on research or clinical findings. Also, as has been our practice in past publications, we list *all* authors of publications wherever possible. We believe that limiting the number of authors of a given publication to a maximum of three is an arbitrary convention presumably intended to save journal space and that does not serve the science community. We hold that all authors are equally important, and they should all be cited.

In addition, we name journals in full. The references should be cited in a way that makes it easy for readers to find them should they wish to do so. Wherever possible, we also provide the Digital Object Identifier (DOI) of publications simplifying online reference retrieval. In most cases, the DOI is all that is needed to find a reference. Unfortunately, a small number of journal publications do not have a DOI. However, in some cases, there is an NIH public access PMC or PMCID number.

Also, we have adopted a numbering system that supersedes the within-journal section number (where those appear) so as to facilitate your access to the information.

Robert Fried, PhD
New York City, NY

Richard M. Carlton, MD
Port Washington, NY

Disclaimer

The information in this book is neither intended to diagnose nor treat any disease, nor is it a substitute for medical guidance. The authors do not propose that anyone who is undergoing treatment for any medical condition under the care of a physician, or any other qualified healthcare provider, should terminate such treatment in favor of any treatment or substance described here.

Rather, where it may seem helpful to adopt a nutrition strategy based on foods or supplements described here, the authors urge the reader to do so only with the advice and the supervision of his or her physician or other qualified healthcare provider.

The information provided here is intended only to educate the reader to what may be available and not to suggest self-treatment. The authors shall not be held liable or responsible for any misunderstanding or misuse of the information contained in this book or for any loss, damage or injury caused or alleged to be caused directly or indirectly by any treatment, action or application of any food or food source discussed in this book.

Acknowledgments

We wish to express our sincere appreciation to Ms. Randy Brem, Senior Editor, Life Sciences and Nutrition, CRC Press/Taylor & Francis Group LLC, for her enthusiastic support of this project. We thank Dr Lynn Nezin for providing the yummy omega-3-rich recipes in Chapter 9. We thank William S. Harris, PhD, FASN, Professor, Department of Internal Medicine, Sanford School of Medicine, University of South Dakota, and Founder and President, Fatty Acid Research Institute, for his help in clarifying a number of very basic issues.

1 What Is the Omega-Factor?

The Lord hath created medicines out of the earth; and he that is wise will not abhor them.

Ecclesiasticus 38:4 (KJV)

1.1 THE MYTH OF THE PALEOLITHIC GOURMET

It is increasingly obvious that the chronic diseases that plague us now, such as hypertension, atherosclerosis, coronary heart disease, obesity and metabolic syndrome, Type 2 diabetes, chronic kidney disease and arthritis, are somehow linked to the foods we consume on a regular basis, independent of how they are processed before they reach our table. And there was a time when it was thought that the main problem with "poor nutrition" was vitamin deficiency. There were vitamin deficiencies, of course, such as beriberi (vitamin B1 deficiency), scurvy (vitamin C deficiency) and rickets (vitamin D deficiency). But these no longer concern us much in modern times, whereas we do implicate nutrition in the chronic disorders that plague us today.

In large measure, we now recognize that loading up on sugars, salt and saturated fats is likely not a great idea, and "health experts" are suggesting alternatives. One of these is the Paleolithic diet, predicated on the proposition that we have distanced ourselves, to our health disadvantage, from the diet of the hunter-gatherers that made up our Paleolithic ancestry.

What was so great about their diet? Among other things, it was said to have the ideal omega-6 to omega-3 fatty acids (FAs) ratio. What are FAs?

FAs are the building blocks of the lipids and fats in the body and in the foods we eat. During digestion, we break down fats into FAs, which can then be absorbed into the blood. FA molecules are sometimes joined together in groups of three, forming a molecule called a triglyceride. Triglycerides are also made in the body from the carbohydrates that we eat. FAs have many important functions in the body, including energy storage. If, for instance, glucose, a type of sugar, isn't available for energy, we can use FAs to fuel the cells instead.

Paleolithic Europe, the Old Stone Age in Europe, encompassed the era from the arrival of the first humans, about 1.4 million years ago until around 10,000 years ago. What is it that it is thought our Paleolithic forebear hunter-gatherers hunted and gathered to eat that was so desirable and nutritious—when they could find it—that we would want it as staple foods today?

Although the diet of people in the Paleolithic era varied by geographic region and availability of foods, most Paleolithic diets would have contained mostly raw meats, some berries, fruits and nuts. No cereals, grains or milk products. And there would have been no vegetables, as we know them, anywhere. Besides, we evolved as meat eaters—the stomach can actually fully digest only meats. That, by the way, is why we look to vegetables for indigestible "fiber."

So, their diet would be more aptly termed "the hunter-scrounger's diet."

Now, omega-6 FAs are found mostly in sunflower, safflower, soy, sesame and corn oils. Walnuts, flaxseed and fish are a good and likely source of omega-3s—so are crickets. Neanderthals living on the shores of Portugal left great mounds of mollusk shells, mostly from clams and mussels. Mollusks are a good source of omega-3s—but not as good as fatty fish. So, it challenges credulity to hold that the foods consumed by people in prehistory is what should be our diet today.

Keep in mind that for all of the toxins, pesticides, saturated fats, salt and sugars in our foods, we are, in fact, on average, living longer. And there lies the real problem, namely that so many of us are living longer but with chronic illnesses, and so many of us are not living as long as we could live because of these illnesses.

What we can do today to correct that disaster cannot depend solely on consuming meat, mussels, blueberries and, oh yes, crickets. What science has found is that a diet rich in both omega-6 and omega-3 FAs is the healthy nutrition that averts chronic illnesses. And what is important—bottom line—is *how much* omega-3s we are getting in the foods we regularly consume. That quantity determines the *Omega-3 Index*, and that index is the key to preventing chronic medical disorders and their consequences, even to reversing them. And that's what this book, *The Omega-Factor*, is all about.

Finally, because we are dealing with a relatively new science of nutrition, and to demonstrate the proven scientific basis of the value of omegas in diet, we have chosen an *evidence-based* presentation: Instead of "we now know that …," we will relate exactly what was found followed by a reference to the scientific journal publication in which it was reported, accessible on the National Library of Medicine (PubMed) website. The citations in the book take the form of a brief synopsis that we stripped of the statistics, science-babble and jargon that usually make up the bulk of scientific journal reports. However, we ask that you pay attention to the word "significant" where it appears, because it is a buzzword from statistics that stands for "these findings are not likely due to chance."

1.2 OMEGA-3 FATTY ACIDS SAVE LIVES

The very popular books that tout diet as a means to good health, youthfulness and longevity have not made a meaningful dent in the latest mortality statistics for the unhealthier, prematurely aging American population. The US Centers for Disease Control and Prevention (CDC), National Center for Health Statistics, in fact recently reported that life expectancy in the United States actually dropped by 1.5 years from 78.8 years in 2019 to 77.3 years in 2020.

This book will show that science has definitively proven that if one's Omega-3 Index, the amount of the omega-3 FAs (eicosapentaenoic acid + docosahexaenoic acid) (EPA + DHA) as measured in the red blood cell membranes, is low, and if one does not begin to incorporate certain foods in the diet right away, one will sooner or later be plagued with cardiovascular and related diseases, age more rapidly and die earlier than might otherwise be the case (1).

Recent medical research has published statistics showing that millions of Americans have a low omega-3 intake, causing widespread omega-3 deficiency which is ultimately responsible for most of the health risks that plague Americans. But we can detail what scientists have more recently found about omega-3 FA-rich foods and food combinations that will slow aging and that will reduce one's risk of all-cause mortality.

Consider these statistics: According to the CDC, coronary heart disease is the most common type of heart disease in the United States. It killed 360,900 people in 2019. About 18.2 million adults in the United States aged 20 and older have coronary heart disease. That's nearly 7%. What's more, adults younger than 65 now account for about 2 in 10 deaths from coronary heart disease. Wouldn't you think that it is time for early action? Well, help is on the way:

If you don't believe us, would you believe the *New England Journal of Medicine*? In 2002, it published the results of a clinical study titled "Blood levels of long-chain n–3 fatty acids and the risk of sudden death" ("n" here stands for omega). In that study, they analyzed the FA composition of whole blood in healthy men without a confirmed history of cardiovascular disease who were participants in the Physicians' Health Study.

The authors, all medical scientists at the Division of Preventive Medicine, Department of Medicine, Brigham and Women's Hospital, Boston, MA, a division of Harvard Medical School, found that consuming the omega-3 FAs found in fish are strongly associated with a reduced risk of sudden death among men without evidence of prior cardiovascular disease.

They report that omega-3 FAs found in fish tend to lower the risk of heart arrhythmias and that dietary supplements of omega-3 FAs may significantly reduce the risk of sudden death among survivors of a prior myocardial infarction (2). This should be wonderful news, especially for those among us who have already survived a heart attack, and who know that they are now at a significantly greater risk of yet another one.

According to the American Heart Association (AHA), each year there are about 335,000 recurrent heart attacks in the United States and about one in five people who have had a heart attack will be readmitted to the hospital for a second one within 5 years (3). That's a daunting prospect. But the evidence is that people with higher levels of omega-3 FAs in their diet are much less likely to succumb to sudden cardiac death than people with lower levels.

This book, *The Omega-Factor*, describes the omega-6/omega-3 ratio, and what it has helped us to understand. It will explain the Omega-3 Index, an evaluation of omega-3 FAs in the body; and it will be a guide to the websites of readily accessible laboratories where, at a reasonable cost, one can find out if there are adequate omega-3 FAs (Omega-3 Index) in the body.

Now, the Mediterranean Diet is said to be one of the healthiest diets in the world. But one can rigidly adhere to a Mediterranean Diet plan and still wind up with an unfavorable omega-6/omega-3 ratio because the food mix chosen may not necessarily supply adequate amounts of omega-3s. Surely all the foods in the Mediterranean Diet plan are "good" foods, but not in random proportion. So, it is the amount of omega-3s that counts.

The Mediterranean Diet has greatly contributed to the long lifespan in Spain—an average life expectancy of 82.8 years. However, what makes it unique is the per capita household consumption of fish that reached 60.8 pounds (lbs) per person, per year. In sharp contrast, the US per capita fish consumption in 2019 hit only 19.2 lbs per person. That's only about 33% of what average citizens of Spain consume. And guess what, fish is one of the best—albeit not the only—source of omega-3 FAs. Now to get a sense of what that means in real life: The US average life expectancy in 2019 (before Covid-19) was 78.8 years, which is four fewer years of life than the 82.8-year average life expectancy in Spain.

So what's the message? Eat more fish and you'll live longer? That's a good start.

Now, the Western Pattern Diet that is also called the Standard American Diet (SAD) is a modern dietary pattern that is typically high in intakes of red meat, processed meat, pre-packaged foods, butter, candy and other sweets, fried foods, conventionally raised animal products, high-fat dairy products, eggs, refined grains, potatoes, corn (and high-fructose corn syrup), along with low intakes of fruits, vegetables, whole grains, pasture-raised animal products, fish, nuts and seeds (5). And it is often washed down with a high-sugar (probably corn syrup) drink. On average, Americans drink about 39 gallons of that stuff each year.

In Spain, on the other hand, a country whose citizens outlive Americans by an average of 4 years, dinner might include fresh fish or seafood, or a portion of roast chicken or lamb with fried potatoes or rice. An omelet and fish with a green salad on the side are also quite common (6). Their diets also supply fats—some animal fats, some vegetable fats—in different quantities. Fats are absolutely necessary to our health. Even basic body cells wither without them.

1.3 FATS—A PRIMER

It is often an uphill battle to try to convince people that dietary fats are an absolute necessity: Fat in skin helps to form vitamin D; vitamin D helps absorb fat—and it is, in fact, the basis of many of our hormones, estrogen, for one.

For example, a clinical study reported in the *Journal of the National Cancer Institute*, titled "Effect of low-fat diet on female sex hormone levels," assigned premenopausal women to a low-fat diet, deriving only 20% of their energy from fat for two months. It was found that the low-fat diet decreased levels of both non-protein-bound estradiol and non-protein-bound testosterone (7). Testosterone, by the way, is the hormone that drives sexual desire in women as well as in men.

But there are good fats and there are harmful fats. For instance, there are polyunsaturated FAs consumed in the diet, such as omega-3 and omega-6 FAs, and these are healthy fats. In contrast there are the saturated fats (so-called because they are "saturated" with hydrogen atoms, due to which they have a solid consistency at room temperature), and on the whole these tend to be unhealthy fats. Saturated fats can be found in a variety of foods, including:

- Animal meat including beef, poultry, pork.
- Certain plant oils such as palm kernel or coconut oil.
- Processed meats including bologna, sausages, hot dogs and bacon.
- Pre-packaged snacks including crackers, chips, cookies and pastries.

These fats are useful in cuisine because they are hard at room temperature and are stable for relatively long periods of time. Also, they don't become rancid as fast as the more liquid, unsaturated fats. However, eating saturated fats raises levels of harmful low-density lipoprotein (LDL), the so-called and inappropriately named "bad cholesterol," that can contribute to plaque buildup along with triglycerides (another type of fatty material).

LDL lipoprotein, i.e., low density lipoprotein, is often called the "bad" cholesterol because it can collect in the walls of our blood vessels causing atherosclerosis and raising our chances of health problems like a heart attack or stroke. More about that in Chapter 4. High levels of this LDL in the diet are harmful. On the other hand, high-density lipoprotein or HDL, the so-called "good cholesterol," discourages plaque buildup.

Monounsaturated fats are typically liquid at room temperature and include:

- Olive, peanut and canola oils.
- Avocados.
- Nuts such as almonds, hazelnuts and pecans.
- Seeds such as pumpkin and sesame seeds.

Polyunsaturated fats are also liquid at room temperature. They include:

- Sunflower, corn, soybean and flaxseed oils.
- Walnuts.
- Flaxseeds.
- Fish oils.
- Canola oil—though higher in monounsaturated fat, it's also a good source of polyunsaturated fat.

To know the chemical difference between mono and poly is not very important. Omega-3 and omega-6 FAs are (poly)unsaturated and those polyunsaturated fats are potentially healthier than monounsaturated fats.

Investigators from the Brigham and Women's Hospital and Harvard Medical School, Boston, MA, reported, in 2010, that replacing foods high in saturated fats with polyunsaturated fat sources reduced the risk of heart disease by 19% (8). In fact, according to the AHA, eating certain polyunsaturated fats can actually decrease total "cholesterol levels" (9).

Mono- and polyunsaturated fats, found in vegetable oils, are all very liquid at room temperature and are unstable, compared to saturated FAs which are solid like lard, butter and tallow. As a consequence, the food industry re-saturates these unsaturated fats by adding back hydrogen—a process called "hydrogenation." Most of the vegetable fats we eat in margarines and other oils are partially hydrogenated to make them less liquid. The more solid the margarine is, the more hydrogenated the fat is, and the less "healthy" it is. The problem with the hydrogenation process is that it makes an unsaturated fat behave more like a saturated fat with all the resultant health problems that come with that. In addition, the hydrogenation process causes the fat molecule to bend from a healthy "cis" configuration into an unhealthy "trans" configuration, and that is why there has been a great effort to encourage Americans to cut down on "trans" fats by limiting their intake of hydrogenated fats and oils (like margarine in particular).

1.4 WHAT IS CHOLESTEROL?

Cholesterol is, per se, not actually a fat, but is a lipid, a substance that does not dissolve in water as it circulates in the bloodstream. It is mostly made by the liver, but we can also get it from foods such as egg yolks, meat and cheeses. Formed by all animal cells, it is an essential structural component of their membranes, a part of the "glue," as it were, that holds their layers together and allows flexibility. The sex hormones, estradiol and testosterone are formed from cholesterol. Estradiol is the strongest of the three naturally produced estrogens and the main estrogen that maintains the reproductive system in women. Steroid hormones (such as cortisol) are also derived from cholesterol.

The molecules that are commonly called "cholesterols," namely HDL, LDL and very-low-density lipoprotein (VLDL), are not different forms of cholesterol. They are actually lipoproteins that carry cholesterol along with other lipids. They are a combination of fat (lipid) and protein. The lipids need to be attached to the proteins so that they can move through the blood. There are at least three different types of lipoproteins.

- Low-density lipoprotein (LDL) is one of the two main lipoproteins. LDL is often called "the bad cholesterol."
- High-density lipoprotein (HDL) is the other main lipoprotein. HDL is often called "the good cholesterol."
- Very-low-density lipoproteins (VLDLs) are particles in the blood that carry triglycerides.

It is when LDL oxidizes, i.e., combines with oxygen, that it initiates atherosclerosis.

1.5 WHAT ARE "TRIGLYCERIDES?"

Triglycerides are the most common type of fat in your body. They are the saturated, monounsaturated and polyunsaturated FAs in the body, and they come from foods, especially butter, oils and other fats most of us consume. They can also come from the extra calories, those that the body does not need right away. The body then changes them into triglycerides and stores that in fat cells. When the body needs energy, it releases the triglycerides. VLDL cholesterol particles transport the triglycerides to our tissues. However, much as we need triglycerides as stored energy, having a high level can raise the risk of heart diseases, such as coronary artery disease.

Because pure cholesterol cannot mix with or dissolve in the blood, the liver packages it with triglycerides and proteins in carriers, lipoproteins. The lipoproteins move this fatty mixture to areas throughout the body.

Foods that contain omega-3 FAs have been found to be very powerful in lowering triglycerides. However, as reported in a number of studies, when omega-3 FAs decrease triglyceride levels, this can elevate the LDL cholesterol (LDL-C) levels (10).

1.6 THE OMEGA-6/OMEGA-3 RATIO

Whereas omega-6 FAs are typically found in foods such as soybeans, corn, safflower and sunflower oils, nuts and seeds, meat, poultry, fish and eggs, the omega-3 FAs are synthesized in phytoplankton (marine plants) and ultimately wend their way up the sea fauna food chain. So, keep in mind that omega-3 FAs are found in concentration in fatty fish, but they are not "made" by the fish. They come from phytoplankton which are plant life, on which zooplankton (primitive animal life) feed. These are then eaten by small fish and the omega-3s work their way up the bigger-fish-eat-the-smaller-fish food chain.

Phytoplankton actually form the base of several aquatic food webs ranging from krill to whales. In a balanced ecosystem, they provide food for a wide range of sea creatures. Also known as microalgae, they are similar to terrestrial plants in that they contain chlorophyll and require sunlight in order to live and grow. Most phytoplankton are buoyant and float in the upper part of the ocean where sunlight penetrates the water. They require inorganic nutrients such as nitrates, phosphates and sulfur which they convert into proteins, fats and carbohydrates.

The two main classes of phytoplankton are *dinoflagellates* and *diatoms*. Dinoflagellates have a whip-like tail, or flagella, with which they move through the water and their body is covered with complex shells. Diatoms also have shells, but they are made of a different substance and their structure is rigid and made of interlocking parts. Diatoms do not rely on flagella to move through the water. Instead, they move with ocean currents.

In a balanced ecosystem, phytoplankton are food for a wide range of sea creatures including shrimp, snails and jellyfish but there is also a dark side to phytoplankton. When there is an overabundance of nutrients, phytoplankton can grow out of control and form harmful algal blooms (HABs). These blooms can produce extremely toxic compounds that have harmful effects on fish, shellfish, mammals, birds and even on people.

Marine mammals are at the top of the food chain and they still play an important role in the diet of Arctic peoples.

The term "Omega Factor" refers to the contribution to health and longevity, and the reduction in health risks and the risk of premature death, of maintaining a diet high in omega-3 FAs that can reflect a favorable omega-6 to omega-3 ratio.

Although much is made of it, that ratio per se is actually of little value to us and it will contribute nothing useful to the management of our health through nutrition. It is not likely that the preparation of our meals would include evaluating the omega-6 and omega-3 constituents of the foods that we are preparing. The omega-6/omega-3 ratio is more an epiphenomenon of anthropology involving assessment of available foods and diet patterns throughout history and mostly prehistory—like the Paleo-diet.

Gathering and eating grubs may not grab us nowadays but they are quite high in omega-3s—all insects are. Crickets, for instance, have as much DHA and EPA as salmon—2.8 grams (g) of omega-3 FAs in 100 g (11). Crickets, anyone? They're considered a plague in most parts of the world, but for a province in Cambodia, the millions of crickets that swarm the plains every year are a cause for celebration. There, crickets are a delicacy, served up deep-fried, crunchy and seasoned.

But what really matters is not that ratio, but how much omega-3s we take in and how much of it we are accumulating in our body.

It has been said that a high omega-6 to omega-3 ratio, such as that in the Western diet thought to be as high as 15:1 or more, is unhealthy and leads to inflammation and to heart disease. While that may be the case, it has been misinterpreted to mean that perhaps one should drastically lower the intake of omega-6s. We know now that this is a mistake and that omega-6s are also important in heart health.

In fact, a study titled "Omega-6 fatty acids and risk for cardiovascular disease," published in 2009 in the journal *Circulation*, proposes consuming at least 5–10% of energy from omega-6 FAs to reduce the risk of coronary heart disease. Such a level of intake is said to be quite safe and may be even more beneficial (as part of a low saturated fat, low-cholesterol diet). It is also reported there that the AHA also supports an omega-6 FA intake of at least 5–10% of energy in the context of other AHA lifestyle and dietary recommendations.

To reduce omega-6 FA intakes from their current levels would be more likely to increase than to decrease the risk of coronary heart disease (12). To achieve a lower ratio, we would increase intake of omega-3s, and not decrease omega-6s. The omega-6 to omega-3 ratio is interesting, in its place, but not helpful and it can even be misleading.

1.7 THE OMEGA-3 INDEX (O3I)

The Omega-3 Index is an actual measure of omega-3 FAs in the body that one can take—no prescription required. There is a number of instances when red blood cells are used to determine body tissue concentration of a particular substance of clinical interest. For instance, routine blood tests may look at the body concentration of magnesium by looking at the concentration in blood serum. But this medium poorly and often incorrectly reflects the magnesium level in our tissues. Alternatively, we can ask our physician to do a red blood cell (RBC) magnesium assay. It is usually

What Is the Omega-Factor?

done on request. By the same token, the O3I is the percentage of EPA plus DHA in red blood cells (erythrocyte)—the cell membrane, actually—revealing the body status of EPA and DHA.

The test, developed by Drs W.S. Harris and C. Von Schacky, was first described in 2004, in the journal *Preventive Medicine*, where they reported that red blood cell FA composition reflects long-term intake of EPA + DHA (the O3I), and that deficiency of these FAs should be considered a new risk factor for death from coronary heart disease (13).

Even though most people don't get sufficient amounts of these nutrients from their diets, and the consequence of that deficiency is now well known to be potentially disastrous, few physicians will automatically test for omega-3 level during routine periodic visits, nor are they likely to tell their patients about any of this.

1.8 OMEGA-6 AND OMEGA-3 FATTY ACIDS

Omega-6 and omega-3 FAs are considered *essential* FAs because we can't make them and we must get them from the foods we consume. Omega-3 FAs include (the terms are hyphenated here to help pronunciation):

- Alpha-lino-lenic acid (ALA) found in plant oils, especially flaxseed.
- Eicosa-penta-enoic acid (EPA) which is found in marine oils.
- Docosa-hexa-enoic acid (DHA) which is also found in marine oils (14).

Omega-6 FAs include:

- Lino-leic acid.
- Gamma-lino-leic acid.
- Ara-chid-onic acids.

The typical Western diet is rich in omega-6 FAs because of the abundance of linoleic acid present in corn, sunflower and safflower oils, the mainstay of American cuisine. On the other hand, omega-3 FAs make up only a small portion of our typical daily dietary fat intake and they are usually obtained from two main dietary sources, fish and plants.

Plant oils from flaxseed, soybean and canola, for instance, contain the omega-3 FA ALA from which our metabolism can also form the omega-3 FAs, EPA and DHA. However, our metabolic conversion of ALA to EPA and DHA is quite inefficient and we make only small amounts of them (15). Only about 5% of the ALA we eat gets converted to EPA, and of that, <1% goes on to produce DHA. The typical US intake of ALA is ~1,500 milligrams (mg) per day, so that would generate about 75 mg of EPA and <1 mg of DHA (4). Our most concentrated food source of EPA and DHA is fatty fish. Fish types and their omega-3 concentrations are detailed in Chapter 8.

When we consume omega-3 and omega-6 FAs, some wind up in cell membranes where they also perform important functions involved in the production of proteins.

The predominance of omega-6 FAs in cell membranes can give rise to pro-inflammatory agents whereas the presence of omega-3 FAs promotes secretion of anti-inflammatory agents, so that there is less of a tendency to inflammation.

It should be noted that omega-6 FAs are also very important to health. In fact, they have also been shown to reduce the risk of coronary heart disease—when taken in the context of a diet low in saturated (animal) fats (16).

The cardioprotective effects of omega-3 FAs include:

Reduced risk or heart arrhythmias (anti-arrhythmic)

- Reduced risk of sudden death.
- Possible prevention of atrial fibrillation.
- Possible protection against ventricular arrhythmias.
- Improvement in heart rate variability.

Reduced risk of atherosclerotic plaque formation (anti-atherogenic)

- Reduction in non-HDL-C levels.
- Reduction in TG and VLDL-C levels.
- Reduction in chylomicrons.*
- Reduction in VLDL and chylomicron remnants.
- Increase in HDL-C levels.
- "Improvement" (increase) in LDL and HDL particle size.
- Plaque stabilization.

Reduced risk of blood clots (antithrombotic)

- Decreased platelet aggregation.
- Improved blood flow.

Anti-inflammatory and endothelial protective effects

- Reduced endothelial adhesion molecules† and decreased leukocyte adhesion receptor expression.‡
- Reduction in pro-inflammatory leukotrienes.§
- Vasodilation.
- Decreased systolic and diastolic blood pressure.

---

* Chylomicrons are large triglyceride-rich lipoproteins produced in red blood cells from dietary lipids, namely, fatty acids and cholesterol.
† These molecules engage with the immune system's white blood cells to mediate regional adhesion and/or migration.
‡ Immune system white blood cells establish transient interactions with the blood vessel inner lining, the endothelium, that allows them to roll along the endothelial surface.
§ Leukotrienes are inflammatory mediators produced in leukocytes, components of the immune system.

1.8.1 OMEGA-3S, OF A TYPE, SAVE LIVES

In 2021, the journal *Nature Communications* reported the outcome of a meta-analysis titled "Blood n-3 fatty acid levels and total and cause-specific mortality from 17 prospective studies." A meta-analysis analyzes the outcome of previously published reports—17 of them, in this case. Here, it is the relationship between blood omega-3 FA levels and total and cause-specific mortality. In a "prospective study," participants are enrolled into the study before they develop the disease or outcome in question.

Over an average of 16 years of follow-up it was found that risk for death from all causes was significantly lower, by at least 15–18%, in the highest vs the lowest quintile* for levels of circulating omega-3 FAs (eicosapentaenoic, docosapentaenoic and docosahexaenoic acids). Similar relationships were seen for death from cardiovascular disease, cancer and other causes. However, no such relationship was observed in connection with levels of ALA, suggesting that it is marine, meaning fish-derived omega-3 FA, that is associated with the lower risk of premature death (17).

1.9 OMEGA-6 FATTY ACIDS

Omega-6 FAs are another type of essential polyunsaturated fatty acids (PUFAs). There are a fair number of them and here are three relevant types:

- Linoleic acid (LA).
- Arachidonic acid (AA, ARA).
- Gamma linolenic acid (GLA).

Omega-6 also has numerous beneficial health functions:

- Helps stimulate skin and hair growth.
- Maintains bone health.
- Regulates metabolism.
- Maintains the reproductive system.

Our body forms substances called "eicosanoids" from omega-6 and omega-3 FAs, and these play an important role in the regulation of inflammation. Eicosanoids formed from omega-6 FAs are pro-inflammatory, while those derived from omega-3 FAs are anti-inflammatory.

It is now believed that the rising incidence of chronic inflammatory diseases such as nonalcoholic fatty liver disease (NAFLD), cardiovascular disease, obesity, inflammatory bowel disease (IBD), rheumatoid arthritis and Alzheimer's disease coincide with a trend in our Western diet to a higher omega-6 to omega-3 ratio. Logically, by increasing the intake of omega-3 FAs in our diet, we can lower the ratio to a healthier

---

* A quintile is a fifth of the range of possible values.

number, and there is evidence that this in turn will translate to a reduction in the incidence of these chronic inflammatory diseases (18).

In another prospective study ranging in duration from 2.5 to 32 years, published in the journal *Circulation* in 2019, it was reported that higher levels of LA predominant in omega-6 FA and AA were significantly associated with lower risks of total cardiovascular disease, death from heart disease and from stroke. The authors concluded that LA and AA may help to prevent cardiovascular disease (19). Likewise, a 7% lower risk of incident cardiovascular disease (CVD) was reported comparing people in the top, and those in the bottom fifth of blood or adipose tissue level of LA (20).

1.10 HOW MEANINGFUL IS THE OMEGA-6 TO OMEGA-3 RATIO?

Supposing that you had some means to determine the "ratio" in your next meal, exactly what should it be? Is there a specific number, or a range of acceptable ratios? Let's turn to experts: The Mount Sinai Hospital (NYC) first serves us a heaped tablespoon of the customary *pablum*: "A healthy diet contains a balance of omega-3 and omega-6 fatty acids." Of course, you would expect that in a "well balanced diet." The site tells us that the Mediterranean Diet may have a more favorable omega-3 to omega-6 FAs balance. Studies show that people who follow a Mediterranean-style diet are less likely to develop heart disease (21). Yes, but what's that ratio and how do we "balance" the food choices to achieve it?

Might Healthline help? Here is what you will find on their website: "Those who follow a Western diet are typically eating way too much omega-6s relative to omega-3s. Many believe this is a serious health problem ... A healthy ratio of omega-6 to omega-3 fatty acids appears to be between 1-to-1 and 4-to-1" (22). And we also learn that between 1960 and 2010, although LA rose dramatically in us humans, it remained the same in chimpanzees. Good to know. If they caught on, they'd outsmart us.

Now, the title of their website is "How to Optimize Your Omega-6 to Omega-3 Ratio." The problem is that you don't know what your ratio is, and they don't tell you how to find out. So much for "optimize."

It has been suggested that we evolved on a diet with a ratio of omega-6 to omega-3 FAs of approximately 1:1. In other words, equal amounts of each type. If you mostly consume a Western diet—so-called Standard American Diet (SAD)—the ratio is more likely 15:1-16:1. Western diets are deficient in omega-3 FAs and have excessive amounts of omega-6 FAs compared with the diet on which humans evolved and their genetic patterns were established.

Before they joined "Western" society and first acquired tooth decay because they could now eat sugar, the Inuit, who we call "Eskimo," had a ratio of 1:4. Seal blubber, their then-principal source of food, holds ca. 24% omega-3 FAs consisting of approximately 9% EPA, 5% decosapentaenoic acid (DPA) and 10% DHA. It has more omega-3s than any fish marine source of omega-3s. Blubber is high in vitamin D and the liver is high in iron and folate. But it is doubtful that seal blubber and liver will ever feature prominently on the dinner plate of even the most dedicated "health nut" here.

1.11 HOW TO FIND OUT OUR OMEGA-3 INDEX (O3I)

Anthropologists tell us that our Paleolithic hunter-gatherer forebears likely had an omega-6 to omega-3 ratio of 1:1. That's a very romantic notion: Nature takes care of its children. If only we listened to Mother Nature. This baseless speculation assumes that these ancestors had the same metabolism and digestive enzymes complex as ours, today, and that their food supply was the same as ours today. There is no reason to assume that, because evolution evolves.

In fact, geneticists tell us that omega-3 and omega-6 FAs that can be obtained directly from food such as fish, or synthesized from vegetable oils, are essential for the development and function of the human brain which, it seems, evolved to its present size and complexity from Paleolithic origins. Such an increase must have caused a greater need for these FAs so as to support a larger brain volume because we use a very large portion of dietary fats, predominantly arachidonic acid (AA) and DHA, to feed the brain. They therefore proposed that a shift in diet, characterized by access to food sources that are rich in essential FAs, must have been initiated about 2 million years ago (23).

It is therefore ludicrous to propose that our diet should match that of forebears whose brain could be supported by that "ideal" 1:1 ratio. What would it have been in the Neanderthal *cuisine* prominently featuring woolly mammoth burger and cranberries? Their brains might have evolved even faster had they thrown in a handful of crickets for lots of FAs. Maybe chimpanzees would be much smarter today if they'd switched from bananas to fish ... or crickets, for that matter.

That said, you can know how much omega-3 your body holds: A number of commercial laboratories provide "home test" kits that evaluate a small finger prick sample of blood for FA composition and return a report to the purchaser. For instance,

> **Omegaquant**
> 5009 W. 12th Street, Suite 8
> Sioux Falls, SD 57106
> Phone: 1-605-271-6917
> Toll-free: 1-800-949-0632
> Fax: 1-800-526-9873
> info@omegaquant.com (https://omegaquant.com/what-is-the-omega-3-index/; accessed January 12, 2022)

If you contact them, they will send you a test kit that you return to them with a drop of blood as instructed. You will then receive a report indicating your O3I (24). They also supply the following information about "risk zones":

> High Risk = less than 4%
> Intermediate risk = 4–8%
> Low risk = more than 8%

The O3I as a risk factor for heart disease was first put forth in 2008 in the *American Journal of Clinical Nutrition* by Dr Bill Harris, who co-invented the O3I test. It gives you a percentage which is a measure of the amount of omega-3 FAs, EPA and DHA in your red blood cell membranes. An O3I of 8% or higher is ideal, the lowest risk zone. If your O3I is in the optimal range, your ratio will be OK—it's all about the denominator. However, most people hover around 5–6% or below. And, unfortunately in the United States, many people are at 4% or below—the highest risk zone.

1.12   THE IMPORTANCE OF THE OMEGA-3 INDEX (O3I)

The typical American diet may contain 10 to 15 times more omega-6 FAs than omega-3 FAs and the per capita consumption of meat by Americans between 2013 and 2019 was 264 lbs. In Greece, it was only 165 lbs. For the same time span, the per capita consumption of vegetables in the United States was 145 lbs and in Greece it was 503 lbs. So back then, the average Greek ate about 450 lbs more vegetables per year than the average American, while the average American ate 100 lbs more of meat per year.

Not surprisingly, the Greek Mediterranean Diet prior to the 1960s had an omega-6 to omega-3 ratio of about 2:1 vs our 15:1. But, the current diet of Greeks has raised that ratio closer to 10:1 with dietary innovations such as *McDonald's* now popular in Greece.

And it will come as no surprise that a Greek medical journal reported recently that by moving away from the Mediterranean Diet, the incidence of cardiovascular "events" is rising in Greece (25). And so, metaphorically, as in that well-known song by Joni Mitchell,

> Don't it always seem to go
> That you don't know what you got 'til it's gone
> They paved paradise and put up a parking lot.

(Joni Mitchell. 1970: *Big Yellow Taxi*)

In 2017, Dr Harris and colleagues published a report titled "The Omega-3 Index and relative risk for coronary heart disease mortality: estimation from 10 cohort studies" in the journal *Atherosclerosis*. The publication related the risk for dying from heart disease to the O3I. The investigators concluded that people with a high Index were 30% less likely to die from coronary heart disease (CHD) than people with a low index. And further, their findings support the concept that an index of less than 4% is in the danger zone; that in the 4–8% range is more consistent with good health, and that >8% is even more ideal (26).

What would the O3I look like in different countries worldwide since it would be a reflection of differences in regional diet patterns? Well, in fact, a map showing regional O3I values does exist (see Figure 1.1).

This map was published in 2016 in the journal *Progress in Lipid Research*. The report title is "Global survey of the omega-3 fatty acids, docosahexaenoic acid and eicosapentaenoic acid in the blood stream of healthy adults." It shows the distribution of the concentration of omega-3 FAs worldwide.

Look for the green areas where the O3I is greater than 8%. You won't find any in the "lower 48." But as this is recent lore, you may note that you won't find any in

What Is the Omega-Factor?

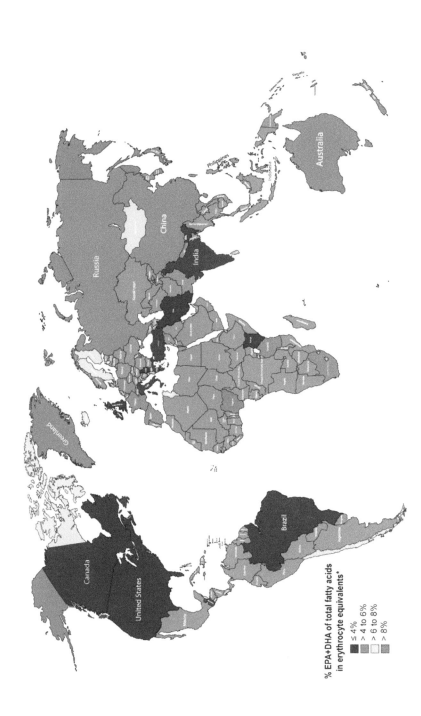

FIGURE 1.1 Global survey of the omega-3 fatty acids in the bloodstream of healthy adults. (From Stark, Van Elswyk, Higgins et al. 2016. *Progress in Lipid Research*, Jul; 63: 132–152. (29). With permission.)

the "Mediterranean" region either since they are rapidly giving up their traditional healthy diet in favor of a *McDonald's* type diet. There's less "paradise" and a growing "parking lot" out there now. What's missing here?

The two green areas shown on the North American continent are Greenland and Alaska. Do you suppose that their population earned such a high O3I by being on a Mediterranean Diet rich in green vegetables? A head of lettuce costs $2.41 in Anchorage, Alaska. In New York City it is $1.40. Now in Greenland, it costs €2.68. That's $3.00. I'll bet they get their omega-3s from fish: In Alaska, statewide, pink salmon costs an average of 30 cents/lb in 2020. Atlantic salmon fillet, the most common type bought in NYC supermarkets, cost an average of $14.99/lb. Lettuce, anyone?

Bottom line, in terms of our body function, what does the O3I actually tell us about our health or risk of death?

1.13 YOUR *HOT-ROD* MITOCHONDRIA

Mitochondria are small structures found in large numbers in most of our cells. They are commonly called the cell "powerhouse" because they are involved in energy production. They form a substance called ATP that transports chemical energy within cells to power metabolism. ATP "captures" chemical energy obtained from the breakdown of food molecules and releases it to fuel other cellular processes. Think of ATP as a battery that can store and then release energy.

Some cells which use a lot of energy (muscles, for instance) have thousands of mitochondria inside, whereas other cells may have only a few hundred. These mitochondria even have their own DNA and protective membrane. They are essentially "cells" within cells that help meet all of the body's basic energy needs. It is well established that mitochondria were originally free-living bacteria that came to reside inside eukaryotic cells, with mutual benefits to their continuing to live there. Well, nothing comes without a price: just as a car has pollutant emission when it runs, mitochondria belch out free radicals. They gulp oxygen and they belch out more oxygen as fractured free radicals.

1.14 THERE'S NO FREE LUNCH

Free radicals are those things that make butter rancid and rust our cars. They can knock chunks out of our DNA and cause cancer. Probably the best-known free radical is oxygen when in certain configurations, the basis for development of most free radicals in the body. Inherently, oxygen is an unstable molecule.

A single oxygen atom has unpaired electrons in its outer orbit. To become stable, two single atoms combine, resulting in the well-known molecule, O_2. But, in metabolism, the O_2 molecule is split, and energy is released. To regain stability—which it is driven to do—the free single oxygen atom, now called an oxygen free radical, free radical for short—seeks out or steals electrons from other available sources. This may result in a bond with dangerous, toxic properties:

Left on the kitchen counter, butter will combine with free radicals to form a new species of butter, i.e., rancid. This combination of free radicals with another substance that now becomes radical is called a Reactive Oxygen Species (ROS). Keep that term in mind because it will come up repeatedly. Scientists don't usually talk about the effect of free radicals because, per se, they don't amount to much until they combine with sugars, proteins or lipids in your body where they wreak havoc: Free radical oxygen can combine with, let's say, lipoproteins in our blood to form the ROS that hardens our arteries and forms atherosclerosis.

So as the mitochondria belch out free radicals, they are at risk of being seriously damaged by those same free radicals because cells have lots of all kinds of fats and there could be an overwhelming outpouring of radicalized ROS. But Nature doesn't miss a trick. The mitochondria can also quench or neutralize these free radicals with antioxidants. Mitochondria make lots of those too and one of the better known is *ubiquinol*. We call it CoQ10. There are several others.

Ordinarily, the quenching function is up to the task. But when there are more free radicals/ROS than can be neutralized and the body battles to fight them off, there is a price to pay: Medicine calls it "oxidative stress," and it is thought to be the very basis of cardiovascular disease… all inflammatory diseases, in fact.

Free radicals and ROS are opposed by antioxidants (next chapter) and, here's the important part: Omega-3 FAs are, first and foremost, antioxidants. And a high O3I is a clue to how well we are using antioxidants to keep oxidative stress at bay. And that is why a high index reduces the risk of premature death from heart disease—by nearly 20%.

Now, regarding slowing aging …

1.15 THE *THREE FATES*

Dr Faust will confirm that nothing short of a pact with the devil will keep us alive forever. Nature sees to that. But Nature is kind. It kills us slowly. We, on the other hand, have the option of speeding up the process and with an omega-3-poor diet, and we can quite effectively accomplish that.

In ancient Greek mythology, life was, metaphorically, an unwinding spool of thread; and three "*Fates*" determined how long the thread would last. Clotho is the Spinner, Lachesis is the (time) allotter and Atropos cuts the thread—of our life—and so determines the moment of death. The ancient Greeks could not know how close they came to biological reality.

If you looked through a microscope into a typical cell in your body, you would see the chromosomes in the nucleus. And, at the end of each chromosome you would see a sort of cap like that at the end of shoelaces that keeps them from unraveling. These caps are called *telomeres*. They keep the chromosomes from unraveling and the DNA from spilling out—which it would otherwise do when the cell divides to replicate.

Figure 1.2 shows that each time a cell divides to replicate, the telomeres become shorter—the *spool* is unwinding—because it passes on shorter telomeres to its "daughter cells." Almost all cells in the body do this. Eventually, the telomeres become so short that the cell can no longer replicate and that spells the end—thanks to Atropos. Now, the faster they do this, the shorter our lifespan.

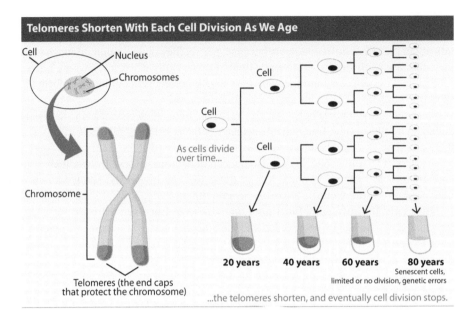

FIGURE 1.2 Each cell replication passes on shorter telomeres to the "daughter cells." (From Elena A Kozyreva; www.antiaging4everyone.com. With permission.)

Omega-3s, as antioxidants, protect telomeres and prevent premature aging. Omega-6s don't accelerate aging, but ROS and inflammation attack our cells, can damage DNA and shorten telomeres thus causing premature aging. Telomere length is linked to exposure to pro-inflammatory substances (cytokines) and oxidative stress, and shorter telomeres portends premature death.

In a study reported in 2013 in the journal *Brain, Behavior and Immunity*, investigators aimed to determine whether omega-3 FA supplementation could lower inflammation. To that end, they chose to examine the telomeres in white blood cells (leukocytes) in healthy sedentary, overweight middle-aged and older adults, who were given:

- 2.5 g/day omega-3 FAs,
- 1.25 g/day omega-3 FAs, or
- Placebo capsules that mirrored the proportions of FAs in the typical American diet.

It was found that supplementation with omega-3 FAs significantly lowered oxidative stress as measured by a predominant lipid biomarker of oxidative stress in humans. It was found to be significantly lower in the omega-3 treatment groups than in the placebo participants group. What's more, telomere length increased significantly with decreasing omega 6:3 ratios, suggesting that lower (which as we learned means healthier) omega-6:omega-3 FA ratios can directly slow down cell aging (27).

In this study, please note that the ratio was lowered/improved by supplementing omega-3s, not by reducing omega-6s, thereby confirming that it is not simply the ratio, per se, that counts.

Even the *Journal of the American Medical Association* (JAMA)—no less—published a report titled "Association of marine omega-3 fatty acid levels with telomeric aging in patients with coronary heart disease." Now these folks with coronary heart disease are displaying shorter telomeres. The investigators reported that: "Each [scientific mathematical metric given] increase in baseline omega-3 fatty acid levels was associated with a 19% decrease in the odds of telomere shortening" (28).

Keep in mind that each time we lose that oxidative stress battle by running short on the antioxidants in omega-3s, it's a win for Atropos.

REFERENCES

1. https://omegaquant.com/ omega-3-index-basic/; accessed 1/7/22.
2. Albert CM, Campos H, Stampfer MJ, Ridker PM, Manson J-AE, Willett WC, and J Ma. 2002. Blood levels of long-chain n-3 fatty acids and the risk of sudden death, *New England Journal of Medicine*, 2002. 46: 1113–1118. https://doi.org/10.1056/NEJM oa012918.
3. https://www.heart.org/en/news/2019/04/04/proactive-steps-can-reduce-chances-of-second-heart-attack; accessed 1/9/22.
4. Plourde M, and Cunnane SC. 2007. Extremely limited synthesis of long chain polyunsaturates in adults: implications for their dietary essentiality and use as supplements. *Applied Physiology, Nutrition and Metabolism*, 32: 619–634. https://doi.org/10.1139/H07-034.
5. Halton TL, Willett WC, Liu, S, Manson JAE, Stampfer M, and FB Hu. (2006) Potato and french fry consumption and risk of type 2 diabetes in women. *The American Journal of Clinical Nutrition*, 83(2): 284–90. https://doi.org/10.1093/ajcn/83.2.284.
6. https://www.thespruceeats.com/meals-and-the-culture-of-spain-3083066; accessed 1/7/22.
7. Ingram DM, Bennett FC, Willcox D, and de Klerk N. 1987. Effect of low-fat diet on female sex hormone levels. *Journal of the National Cancer Institute*, Dec; 79(6): 1225–1229. PMID: 3480374.
8. Mozaffarian D, Micha R, and S Wallace. 2010. Effects on coronary heart disease of increasing polyunsaturated fat in place of saturated fat: a systematic review and meta-analysis of randomized controlled trials. *PLoS Medicine*, Mar 23; 7(3): e1000252. https://doi.org/10.1371/journal.pmed.1000252.
9. https://www.heart.org/en/healthy-living/healthy-eating/eat-smart/fats/polyunsaturated-fat; accessed 1/7/22.
10. Harris WS. 1997. n-3 fatty acids and serum lipoproteins: human studies. *American Journal of Clinical Nutrition*, May; 65(5 Suppl) Suppl: 1645S–1654S. https://doi.org/10.1093/ajcn/65.5.1645S.
11. https://eatsens.com/blogs/news/crickets-are-a-nutritional-powerhouse; accessed 1/11/22.
12. Harris WS, Mozaffarian D, Rimm E, Kris-Etherton P, Rudel LL, Appel LJ, Engler MM, Engler MB, and F Sacks. 2009. Omega-6 fatty acids and risk for cardiovascular disease. *Circulation*, 119: 902–907. https://doi.org/10.1161/ CIRCULATIONAHA.108.191627.
13. Harris WS, and C Von Schacky. 2004. The Omega-3 Index: a new risk factor for death from coronary heart disease? *Preventive Medicine*, Jul; 39(1): 212–220. https://doi.org/10. 1016/j.ypmed.2004.02.030.

14. Nettleton JA. 1995. *Omega-3 fatty acids and health*. New York: Springer.
15. Surette ME. 2008. The science behind dietary omega-3 fatty acids. *Canadian Medical Association Journal*, Jan 15; 178(2): 177–180. https://doi.org/10.1503/cmaj.071356.
16. https://www.cochrane.org/CD 011094/VASC_omega-6-fats-prevent-and-treat-heart-and-circulatory-diseases; accessed 1/10/22.
17. Harris WS, Tintle NL, Imamura F, Qian F, Ardisson Korat AV, Marklund M, Djoussé L, Bassett JK, Carmichael P-H, Chen Y-Y, Hirakawa Y, Küpers LK, Laguzzi F, Lankinen M, Murphy RA, Samieri C, Senn MK, Shi P, Virtanen JK, Brouwer IA, Chien K-L, Eiriksdottir G, Forouhi NG, Geleijnse JM, Giles GG, Gudnason V, Helmer C, Hodge A, Jackson R, Khaw K-T, Laakso M, Lai H, Laurin D, Leander K, Lindsay J, Micha R, Mursu J, Ninomiya T, Post W, Psaty BM, Risérus U, Robinson JG, Shadyab AH, Snetselaar L, Sala-Vila A, Sun Y, Steffen LM, Tsai MY, Wareham NJ, Wood AC, Wu JHY, Hu F, Sun Q, Siscovick DS, Lemaitre RN, Mozaffarian D, and The Fatty Acids and Outcomes Research Consortium (FORCE). 2021. Blood n-3 fatty acid levels and total and cause-specific mortality from 17 prospective studies. *Nature Communications*, 12, 2329. https://doi.org/10.1038/s41467-021-22370-2.
18. Patterson E, Wall R, Fitzgerald GF, Ross RP, and C Stanton. 2012. Health implications of high dietary oOmega-6 polyunsaturated fatty acids. *Journal of Nutrition and Metabolism*, 2012: 539426. https://doi.org/10.1155/2012/539426.
19. Marklund M, Wu JHY, Imamura F, Del Gobbo LC, Fretts A, de Goede J, Shi P, Tintle N, Wennberg M, Aslibekyan S, Chen T-A, de Oliveira Otto MC, Hirakawa Y, Eriksen HH, Kröger J, Laguzzi F, Lankinen M, Murphy RA, Prem K, Samieri C, Virtanen J, Wood AC, Wong K, Yang W-S, Zhou X, Baylin A, Boer JMA, Brouwer IA, Campos H, Chaves PHM, Chien K-L, de Faire U, Djoussé L, Eiriksdottir G, El-Abbadi N, Forouhi NG, Gaziano JM, Geleijnse JM, Gigante B, Giles G, Guallar E, Gudnason V, Harris T, Harris WS, Helmer C, Hellenius M-L, Hodge A, Hu FB, Jacques PF, Jansson J-H, Kalsbeek A, Khaw K-T, Koh W-P, Laakso M, Leander K, Lin H-J, Lind L, Luben R, Luo J, McKnight B, Mursu J, Ninomiya T, Overvad K, Psaty BM, Rimm E, Schulze MB, Siscovick D, Nielsen MS, Smith AV, Steffen BT, Steffen L, Sun Q, Sundström J, Tsai MY, Tunstall-Pedoe H, Uusitupa MIJ, van Dam RM, Veenstra J, Verschuren WMM, Wareham N, Willett W, Woodward M, Yuan J-M, Micha R, Lemaitre RN, Mozaffarian D, Risérus U; For the Cohorts for Heart and Aging Research in Genomic Epidemiology (CHARGE) Fatty Acids and Outcomes Research Consortium (FORCE). 2019. Biomarkers of dietary omega-6 fatty acids and incident cardiovascular disease and mortality: an individual-level pooled analysis of 30 cohort studies. *Circulation*, 139: 2422–2436. https://doi.org/10.1161/CIRCULATIONAHA.118.038908.
20. Sanders TAB. 209. Omega-6 fatty acids and cardiovascular disease. Are we getting closer to the truth? *Circulation*, 139: 2437–2439. https://doi.org/10.1161/CIRCULATIONAHA.119.040331.
21. https://www.mountsinai.org/health-library/supplement/ omega-6-fatty-acids; accessed 1/11/22.
22. https://www.healthline.com/nutrition/optimize-omega-6-omega-3-ratio#TOC_TITLE_HDR_2; accessed 1/11/22.
23. Ameur A, Enroth S, Johansson Å, Zaboli G, Igl W, Johansson ACV, Rivas MA, Daly MJ, Schmitz G, Hicks AA, Meitinger T, Feuk L, van Duijn C, Oostra B, Pramstaller PP, Igor Rudan I, Wright AF, Wilson JF, Campbell H, and U Gyllensten. 2012. Genetic adaptation of fatty-acid metabolism: A human-specific haplotype increasing the biosynthesis of long-chain omega-3 and omega-6 fatty acids. *American Journal of Human Genetics*, May 4; 90(5): 809–820. https://doi.org/10.1016/j.ajhg.2012.03.014.

24. Gupta R, Dhatwalia S, Chaudhry M, Kondal D, Stein AD, Prabhakaran D, Tandon N, Ramakrishnan L, and S Khandelwa. 2021. Standardization and validation of assay of selected omega-3 and omega-6 fatty acids from phospholipid fraction of red cell membrane using gas chromatography with flame ionization detector. *Journal of Analytical Science and Technology*, Aug; 12: 33. https://doi.org/10 .1186/s40543-021-00287-1.
25. Michas G, Karvelas G, and A Trikas. 2019. Cardiovascular disease in Greece; the latest evidence on risk factors. *Hellenic Journal of Cardiology*, Sep–Oct; 60(5): 271–275. https://doi.org/10.1016/j.hjc.2018.09.006.
26. Harris WS, Gobbo LD, and NL Tintle. 2017. The Omega-3 Index and relative risk for coronary heart disease mortality: Estimation from 10 cohort studies. *Atherosclerosis*, Jul; 262: 51–54. https://doi.org/10.1016/j.atherosclerosis.2017.05.007.
27. Kiecolt-Glaser JK, Epel ES, Belury MA, Andridge R, Lin J, Glaser R, Malarkey WB, Hwang BS, and E Blackburn. 2013. Omega-3 fatty acids, oxidative stress, and leukocyte telomere length: A randomized controlled trial. *Brain, Behavior and Immunity*, Feb; 28: 16–24. https://doi.org/10.1016/j.bbi.2012.09.004.
28. Farzaneh-Far R, Lin J, Epel E, Harris W, Blackburn EH, and MA Whooley. 2009. Association of marine omega-3 fatty acid levels with telomeric aging in patients with coronary heart disease. *Journal of the American Medical Association (JAMA)*, Jan 20; 303(3): 250. https://doi.org/10.1001/jama.2009.2008.
29. Stark KD, Van Elswyk ME, Higgins MR, Weatherford CA, and N Salem Jr. 2016. Global survey of the omega-3 fatty acids, docosahexaenoic acid and eicosapentaenoic acid in the blood stream of healthy adults. *Progress in Lipid Research*, Jul; 63: 132–152. https://doi.org/10.1016/j.plipres.2016.05.001.

2 If You Ate What They Ate in Okinawa …

Came from a plant, eat it. Was made in a plant, don't.

—Michael Pollan, author and journalist

2.1 INTRODUCTION

In the last chapter, we explained that some of the foods commonly consumed may contain omega-3 and omega-6 polyunsaturated fatty acids (FAs). Not only is it better for the body to have these in the proper proportion, but what is even more important is how much of the omega-3's eicosapentaenoic acid (EPA) + docosahexaenoic acid (DHA) we are actually getting. That amount can be determined by the *Omega-3 Index* and that is the percentage of omega-3 FAs out of the total of all FAs found in our red blood cell membranes. That's how the lab measures it.

2.2 OMEGA-3s ARE PRINCIPALLY POWERFULLY "ANTIOXIDANTS:" WHY DO WE NEED ANTIOXIDANTS?

The energy that powers our body is generated by our metabolism. Metabolism consists of using oxygen to "burn" food as fuel. This takes place principally in little compartments inside our cells called mitochondria. Mitochondria are the engines that run the cells. The number of mitochondria in a cell coincides with how much energy that cell needs to generate and so, as you would expect, the largest number of mitochondria are found in muscle cells and neurons.

There's no free lunch: In ordinary circumstances, a by-product of your energy metabolism is the fracture, as it were, of oxygen molecules so that they become unstable "free radicals." Just as your car emits exhaust fumes when it is running, your mitochondria belch out free radicals—the more energy created, the more free radicals created. So, oxygen free radicals are formed when an oxygen O_2 molecule breaks into two single atoms, leaving each with only one electron. And, just as the amount of exhaust fumes emitted by a car rises with the speed of the engine, so does the outpouring of free radicals rise as body activity rises (Figure 2.1).

By virtue of their instability, i.e., their tendency to grab an electron from wherever they can get it, these oxygen free radicals will combine in the body with sugars, fats or proteins to form what scientists call "Reactive Oxygen Species" (ROS). Look at it this way: If you leave butter uncovered on the kitchen counter, it will combine with

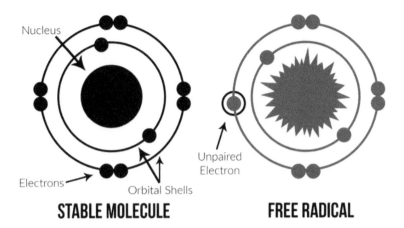

FIGURE 2.1 Free radicals are molecules with an unpaired electron. (From Alexa Ebling. Blondevibe.com. With permission.)

oxygen free radicals in the surrounding air to form a new species of butter, "rancid." A car left outside combines with oxygen free radical in a process we call rusting to form a new species of car, "junk." But the oxygen free radicals that form these new "species" do not come only from the mitochondria, they come from external sources such as tobacco smoke, alcohol, UV sun exposure, pesticides, radiation, pollution and industrial chemicals.

External-source free radicals are termed "exogenous," whereas those that come from mitochondria are "endogenous."

Regardless of their source, free radicals, per se, and ROS compromise the body. They initiate toxic chemical chain reactions both inside our cells where they can damage the outer membrane impairing the integrity of the cell, and in the nucleus where they can chip chunks out of DNA, even shorten telomeres—the string on the spool of life. Outside the body, they assault and damage the cells and structure of our skin.

For all these reasons, ROS are thought to lead to the free radicals/antioxidants imbalance that causes *oxidative stress*, the main culprit in cardiovascular and, as you will see, other all too common chronic inflammatory diseases. Oxidative stress is, in a sense, the price that our body pay to stay in the battle between ROS and antioxidant. Antioxidants are compounds that neutralize free radicals by donating one of their own electrons to free radicals. In so doing, they break a chain reaction that can affect other molecules in the cell and other cells in the body.

2.3 WE HATE THEM BUT WE CAN'T DO WITHOUT THEM

So, just as our body forms ROS, it also forms antioxidants to counter them. There are two types, endogenous antioxidants are formed by our mitochondria, for instance α-tocopherol and ubiquinol. In most but not all cases, exogenous antioxidants are derived from the plants we consume. In fact, they play a major role in plant immune system—the way that plants defend against bacteria, viruses, fungi, etc.

Free radicals can be damaging in the body, but they also serve a very important purpose, and we cannot actually do without them altogether. Among other things, they feature in immune response to bacteria, viruses and other invaders, just as they do in plants. We gain immune defense by eating the plant immune defense: Flaxseed is a powerful antioxidant. It contains minute amounts of cyanogenic glycosides (CGs) which can convert to cyanide when we chew on its seeds. Apple, apricot and cherry pits also contain CGs. It poisons a lot of the bugs, germs and fungi that fancy the seeds when those fall to the ground. That's how come we still have flax ... or apples, or cherries, or apricots.

In our normal consumption of flaxseeds however, there is not enough cyanide produced to be harmful to us. This is explained in Chapter 6. But it's enough to deter plant micro-predators.

Some vitamins such as vitamins C and E, and the minerals copper, zinc and selenium are antioxidants. More about antioxidants later. But keep in mind that "antioxidant" is a chemical process and not a specific aspect of nutrition per se.

We laud the benefits of omega-3 FAs, but while the omega-6s obtained mostly from common cooking oils can, in certain circumstances, be pro-inflammatory, they are also linked to a lower risk of heart disease and stroke. There is every indication that the consumption of at least 5–10% of energy from omega-6 FAs reduces the risk of cardiovascular and heart disease (CHD) relative to lower intakes (1). The health problems begin to stack up when there are few omega-3s. It's the balance that counts.

In context, keep in mind that what both the omega-6 to omega-3 ratio, as well as the Omega-3 Index, i.e., the Omega Factor, tells us the balance between ROS and the available antioxidants to quench them. This balance determines the risk of *oxidative stress* and, consequently, the risk of premature aging and the increased risk of cardiovascular catastrophe.

2.4 THEY LIVE LONGER IN OKINAWA BECAUSE THEY DON'T EAT WHAT YOU EAT

In 2017, the *Journal of the American College of Cardiology* published a scientific report titled "Global, regional, and national burden of cardiovascular diseases for 10 causes, 1990 to 2015." It featured the illustration in Figure 2.2.

Way, way to the right in the middle, there are two small dark blue areas: The one small area that juts out from the coast of China is South Korea and the larger, longer one to the right is Japan. There is a series of barely perceptible dots below Japan. One of them, the closest to Japan, is Okinawa. If you could magnify the image, you would see that the series of dots is also dark blue and there is nothing to differentiate it from Japan, nor from the United States, as far as deaths from cardiovascular disease (CVD) go. In fact, the report does not actually mention Okinawa at all because it is, after all, Japan. But, in terms of the risk of death from CVD, it is far different from Japan proper.

According to the regional colors in Figure 2.2, lifespan in Okinawa and the United States should be about the same because they both fall in the 91 to 220 per 100,000

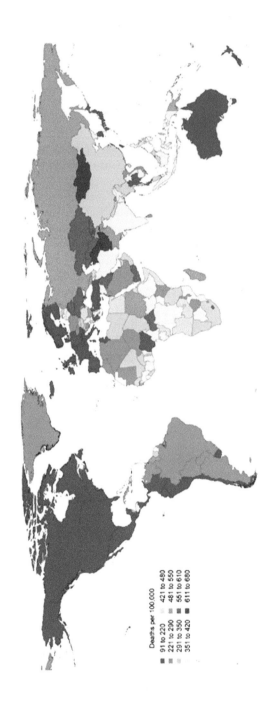

FIGURE 2.2 World map showing the age-standardized rate of deaths from cardiovascular disease in 2015. (From Roth, Johnson, Abajobir et al. 2017. *Journal of the American College of Cardiology*, Jul; 70(1): 1–25. (2). With permission.)

population, dark blue, category. But let's look at some statistics. In 2019 the average Okinawan man lived to 80 years, and the average woman, to 86 years. You may recall that, in the United States in 2019 (before Covid-19), it was 78.8 for men and 81.4 for women. And, for every 100,000 inhabitants, Okinawa had 68 centenarians whereas in the United States it is 3.4. Clearly, there can't be similar rates of deaths from CVD in both those places.

WHY DO OKINAWANS LIVE LONGER ON AVERAGE THAN WE DO?

Have you ever had a friend tell you,

> I saw my doctor yesterday, and she told me that I have all the early warning signs of heart disease. She wrote me a prescription for blood pressure- and cholesterol-lowering medication and then she told me that if I want to prevent it from worsening, I need to eat at least two servings of oily fish like salmon or mackerel twice a week … oh yes, and sweet potatoes.

Fat chance (pun intended).

The basic problem is also the categories used, 91 to 220; 221 to 290, etc. These are too broad. Could that be why, though the rate of death from CVD per 100,000 population is 162 in Japan and 217 in the United States—a difference of 55—yet both are the same dark blue.

We mentioned in the last chapter that the Omega-3 Index and the omega-6 to omega-3 FA ratio are both really about antioxidants. In fact, the source of antioxidants doesn't matter: Okinawans have a low risk of CVD. They eat three servings of fish a week, on average, but it is whole plant foods and not fish that make up the bulk (90%) of their traditional diet. Less than 1% is meat. Their highly anti-inflammatory diet is mostly vegetables and beans, with the most calories coming from purple and orange sweet potatoes that have a 4:1 omega-6 to omega-3 FA ratio.

In addition, sweet potatoes are loaded with the antioxidant *beta carotene*, a carotenoid that the body converts to vitamin A. Purple sweet potatoes are also rich in anthocyanins which are strong antioxidants (see discussion on antioxidants below). To some extent, antioxidants are more or less a feature of all sorts of foods we should consume. Let's take a look at some of these, there's more than just omegas in our meals.

2.5 ANTIOXIDANTS—THE QUICKER PICKER-UPPER

We imagine that our Paleolithic ancestors were the very model of healthy nutrition. They hunted and they gathered in a pristine paradise stocked with a wide variety of healthy foods. So, how come they vanished?

Didn't Darwin tell us that the "fittest" survive? As hunter gatherers, their diet must have been mostly plant, seed, nut and fruit-based—no cola, no canned or otherwise processed food, no margarine—and some red meat … now and then, a fat fish that flopped up onto the shore. So, let's assume that science is right and that they were noted for a high antioxidant diet; in fact, it is also said that their omega-6 to omega-3 ratio may have been 1:1—but not great for brain development, we are told. Ours is said to be closer to 15:1, great for brain development, but not great for reducing the risk of heart disease.

So, we need antioxidants to ward off free radicals and ROS and we've identified four major antioxidant mechanisms that help us to cope with free radicals:

1. They can rid us of metal ions such as iron, zinc and copper.
2. They scavenge and quench free radicals and ROS.
3. They can end chain reactions by free radicals.
4. They can repair damage caused by free radicals and ROS.

2.6 THE ANTIOXIDANTS THE BODY MAKES

We call the antioxidants our body makes "endogenous antioxidants." There is a fair number of endogenous antioxidants, but these five are the major ones:

- Glutathione (GSH).
- Superoxide dismutase (SOD).
- Catalase (CAT).
- Glutathione peroxidase (GPx).
- *Alpha*-lipoic acid.

We get others called "exogenous antioxidants" from the foods we consume, including most of the vitamins that our body needs. By the way, our Paleolithic ancestors, stemming from Africa, did not need sunscreen to protect them from the free radicals in UV sun rays. Nature provided them with an endogenous antioxidant in the form of a skin pigment called *eumelanin*, which is an antioxidant.

EXOGENOUS ANTIOXIDANTS INCLUDE:

- Vitamin C (ascorbic acid/ascorbate) found in bell peppers, strawberries, kiwi, Brussels sprouts, broccoli.
- Vitamin E (tocopherol, tocotrienol) found in vegetable oil, nuts and seeds.
- Carotenoids (alpha-carotene, beta-carotene, zeaxantin, lutein, lycopene, beta-cryptoxantin, etc.) found in orange and red vegetables and fruits (carrots, tomatoes, apricots, plums) and leafy vegetables (spinach, kale).
- Polyphenols (flavonols, flavanols, anthocyanins, isoflavones, phenolic acid) found in fruits (apples, berries, grapes), vegetables (celery, kale, onions), legumes, (beans, soybeans), nuts, wine, tea, coffee, cocoa.
- Trace elements (selenium, zinc) found in seafood, meat, whole grain.

Polyphenols including phenolic acids and flavonoids in concentrations in fruits and vegetables are the most abundant class of food-borne antioxidants. However, to work well for us in our body, some require additional "co-factors" for absorbability.

2.6.1 The Antioxidant Paradox

As you will see, it is how much omega-3 FA we get in our diet that is really important. Just so, it is the balance of free radicals and antioxidants that counts. Our body actually needs free radicals and ROS in our battle against cancer and against infections, for one thing. For instance, the white blood cells, part of our immune system, actually shoot out free radicals at bacteria, viruses and other interlopers. And, ordinarily, barring certain diseases that increase their output and swamp us—Covid-19 "cytokine storm" for one—they would not overwhelm our endogenous antioxidants. By the same token, it is not a great idea to overdo antioxidants either.

While on the one hand, in high concentration, ROS are toxic, potentially life-threatening molecules, on the other hand, at low concentrations, ROS are very important to the way our body functions. They are said to be "signaling molecules" which means that they are messengers to various cells to initiate some vital activity. And they also play a crucial role in the regulation of immune responses because they promote antioxidant defense mechanisms (3). One research team cited ROS as "double-edged swords" in a report, in 2002, in the journal *Human and Experimental Toxicology* (4).

The balance between oxidant (free radical) production and antioxidant protection is believed to be critical in maintaining healthy biological systems. There is also a cooperative action between endogenous and exogenous antioxidants that maintains the balance between free radicals and antioxidants. In fact, in grazing animals, it is par for the course. To that end, we have vitamins such as C, E and carotenoids. Polyphenols, by the way, are better at protecting us than vitamin C. These vitamins are, therefore, antiviral, anti-inflammatory, antiallergenic and anti-aging as well (5).

ROS may also play a role in signaling production of different growth factors. This conclusion is supported by the hypothesis that decreased levels of ROS may lead to degenerative diseases, generating an interesting concept that ROS must be regulated, but not eradicated—"taking the bull by the horns," as they say.

2.7 RESVERATROL FOR WHAT AILS YOU

Resveratrol is said to be abundant in red wine … more in some like certain Pinot Noirs than in others. Resveratrol comes in two forms: *Trans*-Resveratrol and *Cis*-Resveratrol. Trans-Resveratrol is the active form of resveratrol and in concentration—in research studies—it has proven to be antioxidant and helpful in all sorts of medical conditions ranging from protecting the cardiovascular system and neurological function, to fighting cancer.

But, for one thing, it isn't actually abundant in a typical glass of wine that most are likely to be drinking. Furthermore, it is fragile and easily deactivated by exposure to light or heat (6). The success in clinical studies comes from the application of the *trans* form in clinical dosages far exceeding what can be found in a couple of glasses of Pinot Noir—minus the alcohol. You are not likely to get that with your "after dinner," or served at a cocktail party. Furthermore, even "moderate consumption" of wine may not really contribute to health. Consuming alcohol leads to the formation of ROS.

2.8 WHAT IS ORAC? HOW MUCH DO WE NEED?

Apparently, antioxidants can prevent premature aging and significantly reduce the risk of a fatal heart attack. So, wouldn't it be good to know just how antioxidant the antioxidants we are regularly consuming really are? Or, better yet, how antioxidants are the foods we commonly consume?

Writing in the journal *Free Radical Biology and Medicine*, in 1993, three researchers from the Agricultural Research Service (ARS) of the US Dept of Agriculture (USDA) reported that they developed a relatively simple, sensitive and reliable method of measuring how well antioxidants in the blood can eliminate oxygen free radicals. They called it the Oxygen Radical Absorbance Capacity—"ORAC" for short—and it is a test tube analysis that measures the total antioxidant power of foods (and any other chemical substance) (7).

The laboratory method for obtaining ORAC units is based on the comparison of a test sample to the net antioxidant protection of a standard quantity of a water-soluble analog of vitamin E called *Trolox*. So, ORAC assesses the antioxidant capacity of any substance by comparing it to a known antioxidant.

There's another term it helps to know, *TBARS*. TBARS is a substance whose concentration can be used to assess the damage done by ROS. It is measured as the concentration of one of their by-products—a kind of chemical damage signature. In addition, when lipids combine with oxygen, i.e., oxidize—to our health disadvantage—they can decompose and in the process form various other nasty reactive by-products. One of these is called *malondialdehyde*, MDA for short.

Concentration of TBARS and MDA are used by scientists to assess the concentration of ROS in our tissues and if they can reduce them with antioxidants, they can determine the effectiveness of those antioxidants. These are complicated laboratory procedures, and they are not readily available to us to estimate the outpouring of free radicals and the efficacy of both the antioxidants our body makes to counter them plus those we add in diet.

So, we have to rely on the guidelines reported in medical journals by scientists who grapple with TBARS and MDA which they measure in living cells in glass dishes and, more often than not, in fat rats: they can watch fats oxidize lipids, the TBARS and MDA accumulate, and then add antioxidants one by one to reduce ROS. Voila! A list of antioxidants ranked by efficacy—ORAC.

So, ORAC is a number that represents trillions and trillions of free radicals zapped into behaving themselves. The problem, as you will see, is that it says nothing specific about health. So, "What do we learn from this?" one may reasonably ask.

For one thing, if we didn't know how damaging air pollution is, we learn that elevated levels of MDA in urine tells us just how severely that air pollution causes oxidative stress (8). We also learn that daily smokers have greater elevated concentrations of blood MDA than nonsmokers, and so also do those people who are simply exposed to cigarette smoke. And, by the way, weekly alcohol consumption also raises MDA (9).

ROS can cause oxidative stress that can kill us "down the road." But, in certain circumstances, they can kill us right quickly. One such circumstance is *sepsis*. Sepsis occurs when chemicals (cytokines) released in the bloodstream to fight an infection trigger inflammation throughout the body. This can cause a cascade of changes that damage multiple organ systems, leading them to fail, sometimes even resulting in death. This is akin to the "cytokine storm" that can kill Covid-19 sufferers.

If one were to develop sepsis, the concentration of TBARS in urine can accurately predict the likelihood of surviving or dying. A study published in the journal *Medicine*, in 2020, reported that the concentration of TBARS can actually be used to accurately predict fatality in sepsis (10). So, we can measure the concentration of free radicals—albeit indirectly—as ORAC. And, when these free radicals combine with sugars, fats and TBARS and MDA.

What's more, we can use TBARS and MDA to tell us the severity of metabolic stress and, in the extreme case, how likely it is to kill us quickly. And, by the way, it's the ROS generated by the microbes that kill us, not the microbes themselves.

2.9 NO GOOD DEED GOES UNPUNISHED

In February 1999, the *Human Nutrition Research Center on Aging*, a branch of the Agriculture Research Service (ARS) of the US Department of Agriculture (USDA), announced that "High-ORAC Foods May Slow Aging." What does this actually mean? (11). It means that not only is measuring the *oxygen radical absorbance capacity* (ORAC) of foods now feasible, but it tells us, in a way, that the foods with a high ORAC number may actually help us to avert accelerated aging. ORAC can tell us a great deal about omega-3 FAs as well.

The report went on to state that studies of animal and human blood show that foods that score high in their ORAC antioxidant analysis may protect cells and organelles from oxidative damage—"organelles" like mitochondria. What's more, eating plenty of high ORAC-unit fruits and vegetables, such as spinach and blueberries, may help slow aging: "If these findings are borne out in further research, young and middle-aged people may be able to reduce risk of diseases of aging — including senility — simply by adding high-ORAC foods to their diets," so said ARS Administrator, Floyd P. Horn.

Their studies showed that eating "plenty" of high ORAC-unit foods raised the antioxidant power of human blood by 10–25%. "It may be that combinations of nutrients found in foods have greater protective effects than each nutrient taken alone," said Guohua (Howard) Cao, a physician and chemist who developed the ORAC assay.

Then, in November 2007, Rosaline M. Bliss, also from the ARS, released a report titled "Data on food antioxidants aid research" (12). This report included ORAC unit values of 277 selected foods, some shown in Figure 2.3, and it stated that the database can be used to help guide ongoing research into how antioxidants may contribute to health benefits.

For example, many fruits and vegetables are known to be good sources of antioxidant vitamins, such as E, C and beta carotene, a form of vitamin A. But these natural foods also contain other compounds collectively known as *phytonutrients* that may contribute to health and so it is not entirely clear how much is the contribution of

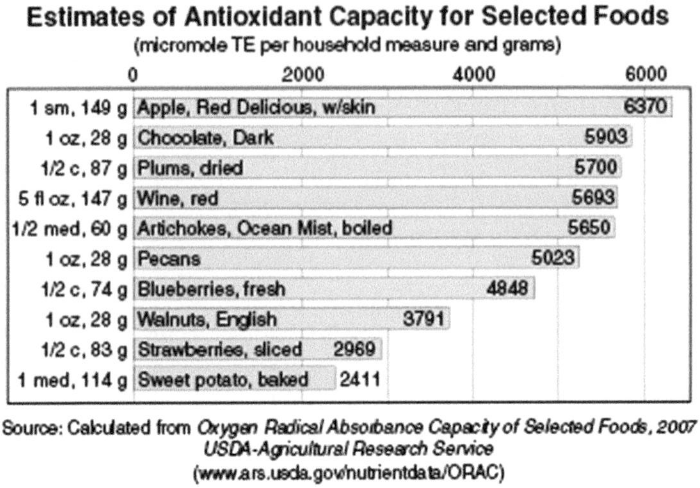

Estimates of Antioxidant Capacity for Selected Foods
(micromole TE per household measure and grams)

Measure	Food	Value
1 sm, 149 g	Apple, Red Delicious, w/skin	6370
1 oz, 28 g	Chocolate, Dark	5903
1/2 c, 87 g	Plums, dried	5700
5 fl oz, 147 g	Wine, red	5693
1/2 med, 60 g	Artichokes, Ocean Mist, boiled	5650
1 oz, 28 g	Pecans	5023
1/2 c, 74 g	Blueberries, fresh	4848
1 oz, 28 g	Walnuts, English	3791
1/2 c, 83 g	Strawberries, sliced	2969
1 med, 114 g	Sweet potato, baked	2411

Source: Calculated from *Oxygen Radical Absorbance Capacity of Selected Foods, 2007* USDA-Agricultural Research Service (www.ars.usda.gov/nutrientdata/ORAC)

FIGURE 2.3 Estimates of antioxidant capacity for selected foods. (From US Department of Agriculture Research Service. 2004. USDA National Nutrient Database for Standard Reference, Release. Nutrient Data Laboratory Home Page, www.ars.usda.gov/nutrientdata.)

their antioxidant properties. Nevertheless, there had initially been a recommendation by the USDA of a minimum of 5,000 ORAC units per day.

Then, the USDA dramatically reversed its position on recommending ORAC because there seemed to them no way to avoid its abuse in marketing health foods and related products. And so, in 2010, ARS issued a repudiation of ORAC, titled "Oxygen radical absorbance capacity (ORAC) of selected foods, release 2 (2010)." It stated, in essence, that there is "mounting evidence that the values indicating antioxidant capacity have no relevance to the effects of specific bioactive compounds, including polyphenols on human health"—that we don't completely understand how bioactive compounds thought to prevent or ameliorate various chronic diseases such as cancer, coronary vascular disease, Alzheimer's and diabetes actually work; or, for that matter how antioxidants really work.

Furthermore, the report claimed—erroneously by the way—that there is no evidence that the beneficial effects of polyphenol-rich foods can be attributed to the antioxidant properties of these foods. For these reasons the ORAC table previously available on their website disappeared. It was argued that no systematic peer-reviewed clinical studies had shown that a given ORAC unit value, or range of values, provides any health benefit or reverses illness.

But in fact, the benefit of antioxidants had been repeatedly reported in human participants in clinical studies. In a report titled "Free radicals, antioxidants and functional foods: impact on human health," published in the journal *Pharmacognosy Review* in 2010, the authors stated that "Antioxidants prevent free radical induced tissue damage by preventing the formation of radicals, scavenging them, or by promoting their decomposition" (13). If you enter "benefits of antioxidants" on the PubMed (government medical library) website, you will be served with 44,148 scientific journal articles from which to choose.

In support of ORAC, the journal *Food Chemistry* reported a study in 2009 comparing ORAC and another measure of antioxidant activity related to Trolox, the vitamin E thing, to measure antioxidant capacity of milk, orange juice and a milk/orange juice combination. It was indeed found that ORAC is an accurate way to measure food antioxidant capacity (14).

But it must be admitted in all fairness that there is no indication that a better assessment of antioxidant capacity of foods says anything about their contribution to better health or to combating illness other than that it is better than nothing. However, a recent clinical study published in the *Nutrition Journal* reported that dietary total antioxidant capacity is inversely related to a marker of inflammation, C-Reactive Protein (CRP), in young Japanese women (15).

There seems to be little disagreement about the beneficial effects of certain antioxidants. It remains to be seen whether a unit-value such as ORAC can be a helpful benchmark for measuring the health benefits of certain foods. ORAC at present tells us little more than that a given ORAC unit value represents more or less antioxidant free-radical-absorbing capacity than another ORAC unit value. For example, 1,800 ORAC units is twice 900. But we can't say that 1,800 units is twice as beneficial to health as 900 units. We also don't know what the lowest ORAC unit value is that has any health benefits, or what the highest unit value is that has adverse—even toxic—effects.

That said, curiously, the *USDA Database for the Oxygen Radical Absorbance Capacity (ORAC) of Selected Foods, Release 2* (2010) somehow reappeared on the internet and can be accessed at: http://www.orac-info-portal.de/download/ORAC_R2.pdf.

Here is a link to a list of ORAC values for foods that contain phytochemicals: https://www.phytochemicals.info/list-orac-values.php. Phytochemicals are what provide the aroma, flavor and color to vegetables and fruits. These chemicals are biologically active, and they help the plants fight off infection, disease and invasion ... in us also.

Keep in mind that a high ORAC unit food may be more "antioxidant" than a low ORAC unit food, but that there is no way that we can interpret ORAC unit value in any more meaningful terms. Furthermore, there is no way to determine what one's antioxidant needs are at any given moment, and what ORAC unit value food(s) would satisfy that need. That said ...

2.10 IT TAKES 2 POUNDS OF BLUEBERRIES TO GET THE ORAC OF 100 GRAMS OF FLAXSEED

ORAC was a good start at evaluating the *potential* health benefits of specific foods but, in the end, it is too abstract for day-to-day application. For instance, 100 grams (g) of blueberries has 2,400 ORAC units, while 100 g of flaxseeds has 19,600. If you were hell-bent on ORAC, you'd have to consume more than eight times 100 g of blueberries to get the equivalent ORAC value of 100 g of flaxseed (about 14 tablespoons) ... almost 2 pounds (lbs) of blueberries—more than 5 cups.

Fatty fish, recommended as a healthy meal with high omega-3 antioxidants, has a lower ORAC value than iceberg lettuce, which is found to have 1,400% more antioxidants than salmon.

By the way, if one is serving children those wonderful chock-full-of-antioxidant blueberries with their cereal and a tall glass of that wonderful, healthful milk, it might be worth knowing that scientists have shown that "The ingestion of blueberries in association with milk ... impairs the in vivo antioxidant properties of blueberries and reduces the absorption of caffeic acid" (16). Caffeic acid is present in all plants, including vegetables, fruits, herbs, coffee beans, plant-based spices and others that we eat and drink. It is anti-inflammatory and antioxidant.

And, yes, ORAC was, and still is, abused in marketing the health benefits of some food products. On the other hand, ORAC turned out to be a useful way to find out how antioxidant the omega-3 and omega-6 FAs actually are. A number of studies show this to be the case. For instance, all the breast cancer patients undergoing chemotherapy in a clinical study published in the *Journal of Medical Case Reports*, in 2015, showed a significant increase in ORAC values after omega-3 FA supplementation (17).

Now, walnuts have both omega-3 and omega-6 FAs and they are very high in the omega-6s. Walnuts and fatty fish contain high amounts of polyunsaturated FAs. They also contain antioxidants that likewise contribute to the reduction of cardiovascular disease. So, the purpose of a clinical study published in the *Journal of the Medical Association of Thailand* in 2012, was to compare the effects of walnuts and fatty fish (as measured by plasma and urine ORAC values). It was found that measures of ORAC were significantly higher in the walnut diet compared with a fish diet and a control diet. Moreover, the ORAC for the food itself was significantly higher in the walnut diet compared with the fish and the control diet. The investigators suggested that because walnuts have a large antioxidant capacity, they should be included in the daily diet to maintain an antioxidant status in the body (18). This study provides a clue to why omega-6s are cardioprotective—it's the antioxidants.

Here you have walnuts high in omega-6s and ORAC at 13,541 per 100 g, and fish low on ORAC value, but high in omega-3s. Three ounces (ca. 0.85 g) of cooked Atlantic farmed salmon holds 1.24 g of DHA and 0.59 g of EPA. You probably didn't think that there is such a thing as a fish and walnut dish. Guess again: check out:

Walnut-crust ginger salmon (https://www.tasteofhome.com/recipes/walnut-crusted-ginger-salmon/(accessed 6.12.22)) and there's lots more where these came from.

The USDA, ARS, FoodData Central, 2019, lists "ALA, EPA, and DHA Content of Selected Foods" (https://ods.od.nih gov/ factsheets/Omega3FattyAcids-HealthProfessional/; accessed January 23, 2022). Here one can see that flaxseed has 7.26 g of alpha-linolenic acid per 100 g, and that it has no EPA or DHA per se.

There is another useful website: The NutritionData website (https://nutritiondata.self. com/foods-009140000000141000000.html?maxCount=138; accessed January 23, 2022) lists "Foods highest in Total Omega-3 fatty acids, and lowest in Total Omega-6 fatty acids."

Now, if one were to decide that the Okinawans have a good thing going, what's on the menu? Here is what their meals consist of: Unlike other Japanese, Okinawans consume very little rice. Instead, their main source of calories is the sweet potato followed by whole grains, legumes and fiber-rich vegetables. By the way, sweet potatoes are also low in lectins, naturally occurring proteins that are found in most plants. Some foods that contain higher amounts of lectins include beans, peanuts, lentils, tomatoes, potatoes, eggplant, fruits and wheat and other grains. They are indigestible and can actually harm the gut, but cooking can reduce their concentration and effects to a limited extent.

The traditional diet in Okinawa consists mainly of root vegetables such as sweet potatoes, green and yellow vegetables, soybean-based foods and medicinal plants such as *Ryukyu yomogi* (Okinawan mugwort), *fuchiba* (felon herb), *seronbenkei* (air plant), *chomeiso* (long life plant) and *hippazu*, an Okinawan pepper. Marine foods, lean meats, fruit, garnishes and spices, tea and alcohol are also moderately consumed.

There are many similarities between the Okinawan diet and the traditional Mediterranean Diet, DASH diet and Portfolio diet. All these dietary patterns are associated with reduced risk for cardiovascular disease, among other age-associated diseases. Overall, the important shared features of these healthy dietary patterns include a high intake of unrefined carbohydrates, moderate protein intake with emphasis on vegetables/legumes, fish and lean meats as sources, and a healthy fat profile (higher in mono/polyunsaturated fats, lower in saturated fat; rich in omega-3s).

The healthy fat intake is likely one way for reducing inflammation[*] and optimizing healthy blood lipids. Furthermore, a lower caloric density of plant-rich diets results in lower caloric intake with concomitant high intake of phytonutrients and antioxidants. Other shared features include low glycemic load,[†] less inflammation and oxidative stress. All in all, this may reduce the risk of accelerating chronic age-associated diseases and it may promote healthy aging and longevity.

A report was published in 2014 in the journal *Mechanisms of Ageing and Development*, titled "Healthy ageing diets other than the Mediterranean: A focus on the Okinawan diet." It described the Okinawan diet to mainly consist of:

- Vegetables (58–60%): Sweet potato (orange and purple), seaweed, kelp, bamboo shoots, daikon radish, bitter melon, cabbage, carrots, Chinese okra, pumpkin and green papaya.
- Grains (33%): Millet, wheat, rice and noodles.
- Soy foods (5%): Tofu, miso, natto and edamame.

---

[*] In a later chapter, we will show that chronic inflammation is a key feature of all chronic health hazards ranging from coronary artery disease to glaucoma.

[†] The Glycemic Index (GI) ranks carbohydrate foods according to the speed at which they cause blood glucose levels to rise and fall. The Glycemic Load (GL) is calculated by multiplying the GI of the food by the amount of carbohydrate per serving and then dividing by 100.

- Meat and seafood (1–2%): Mostly white fish, seafood and occasional pork—all cuts, including organ meats.
- Other (1%): Alcohol, tea, spices and dashi (broth).

Jasmine tea is consumed liberally and antioxidant-rich spices like turmeric are common (19).

The Okinawa diet is not a well-kept secret. Though you don't hear much about it, there are a number of books that describe it. There's a whole page of titles on Google.

Finally, a note of caution: Okinawans consume a considerable amount of seaweed. Even three times the amount of seaweed, i.e., nori (the type wrapping sushi), wakame and those "sea grapes," as do mainland Japanese. Seaweed is quite high in iodine and excess consumption can lead to health problems.

2.10.1 Caveat

First, excess iodine consumption can lead to Hashimoto's disease, an immune disorder. Second, iodine consumed in seaweed and other iodine-rich food will rapidly cause your blood sugar to spike. This is a strong word of caution to those of you with Type 2 diabetes.

REFERENCES

1. Harris WS, Mozaffarian D, Rimm E, Kris-Etherton P, Rudel LL, Appel LJ, Engler MM, Engler MB, and F Sacks. 2009. Omega-6 fatty acids and risk for cardiovascular disease. A science advisory from the American heart association nutrition subcommittee of the council on nutrition, physical activity, and metabolism; Council on cardiovascular nursing; and council on epidemiology and prevention. *Circulation*, 119: 902–907. https://doi.org/10.1161/CIRCULATIONAHA. 108.191627.
2. Roth GA, Johnson C, Abajobir A, Abd-Allah F, Abera SF, Abyu G, Ahmed M, Aksut B, Alam T, Alam K, Alla F, Alvis-Guzman N, Amrock S, Ansari H, Ärnlöv J, Asayesh H, Atey TM, Avila-Burgos L, and C Murray. 2017. Global, regional, and national burden of cardiovascular diseases for 10 causes, 1990 to 2015. *Journal of the American College of Cardiology*, Jul; 70(1): 1–25. https://doi.org/10.1016/ j.jacc.2017.04.052
3. Valko M, Leibfritz D, Moncol J, Cronin MTD, Mazur M, and J Telser. 2007. Free radicals and antioxidants in normal physiological functions and human disease. *International Journal of Biochemistry and Cell Biology*, 39(1): 44–84. DOI: 10. 1016/j.biocel.2006.07.001.
4. Martin KR, and JC Barrett. 2002. Reactive oxygen species as double-edged swords in cellular processes: low-dose cell signaling versus high-dose toxicity. *Human and Experimental Toxicology*, Feb; 21(2): 71–75. DOI: 10.1191/0960327102ht213oa.
5. Pandey KB, and I Rizvi. 2009. Plant polyphenols as dietary antioxidants in human health and disease. *Oxidative Medicine and Cellular Longevity*, Nov–Dec; 2(5): 270–278. DOI: 10.4161/oxim.2.5.9498.
6. Vitaglione P, Sforza S, Galaverna G, Ghidini C, Caporaso N, Vescovi PP, Fogliano V, and R Marchelli. 2005. Bioavailability of trans-resveratrol from red wine in humans. *Molecular Nutrition and Food Research*, May; 49(5): 495–504. DOI: 10.1002/mnfr.200500002.
7. Cao G, Alessio HM, and RG Cutler. 1993. Oxygen-radical absorbance capacity assay for antioxidants. *Free Radical Biology & Medicine*, Mar; 14(3):303–311.

8. Gong J, Zhu T, Kipen H, Wang G, Hu M, Ohman-Strickland P, Lu S-E, Zhang L, Wang Y, Zhu P, Rich DQ, Diehl SR, Huang W, and JJ Zhang. 2013. Malondialdehyde in exhaled breath condensate and urine as a biomarker of air pollution induced oxidative stress. *Journal of Exposure Science and Environmental Epidemiology*, May-Jun; 23(3): 322–327. DOI: 10.1038/jes.2012.127.
9. Nielsen F, Mikkelsen BB, Nielsen JB, Raun Andersen HR, and P Grandjean. 1997. Plasma malondialdehyde as biomarker for oxidative stress: reference interval and effects of life-style factors. *Clinical Chemistry*, 43; 7: 1209–1214. DOI:10.1093/CLINCHEM/43.7.1209.
10. Hsiao SY, Kung C-T, Su C-M, Lai Y-R, Huang C-C, Tsai N-W, Wang H-C, Cheng B-C, Su Y-J, Lin W-C, Chiang Y-F, and C-H Lu. 2020. Impact of oxidative stress on treatment outcomes in adult patients with sepsis. A prospective study. *Medicine*, Jun 26; 99(26): e20872. DOI: 10.1097/MD.0000000000020872.
11. McBride J. Feb. 1999; http://www.ars.usda.gov/is/pr/1999/990208.htm.
12. Bliss RM. 2007; http://www.ars.usda.gov/is/pr/2007/ 071106.htm.
13. Lobo V, Patil A, Phatak A, and N Chandra. 2010. Free radicals, antioxidants and functional foods: Impact on human health. *Pharmacognosy Review*, Jul–Dec; 4(8): 118–126. DOI: 10.4103/0973-7847.70902.
14. Zulueta A, Esteve MJ, and A Frígola. 2009. ORAC and TEAC assays comparison to measure the antioxidant capacity of food products. *Food Chemistry*, 114: 310–316.
15. Kobayashi S, Murakami K, Sasaki S. Uenishi K, Yamasaki M, Hayabuchi H, Goda T, Oka J, Baba K, Ohki K, Watanabe R, and Y Sugiyamama. 2012. Dietary total antioxidant capacity from different assays in relation to serum C-reactive protein among young Japanese women. *Nutrition Journal*, Oct 30; 11: 91. DOI: 10.11 86/1475-2891-11-91.
16. Serafini M, Testa MF, Villaño D, Pecorari M, van Wieren K, Azzini E, Brambilla A, and G Maiani. 2009. Antioxidant activity of blueberry fruit is impaired by association with milk. *Free Radical Biology and Medicine*, Mar 15; 46(6): 769–774. DOI: 10.1016/j.freeradbiomed.2008.11.023.
17. Mansara P, Ketkar M, Deshpande R, Chaudhary A, Shinde K, and R Kaul-Ghanekar. 2015. Improved antioxidant status by omega-3 fatty acid supplementation in breast cancer patients undergoing chemotherapy: a case series. *Journal of Medical Case Reports*, 9: 148. DOI: 10.1186/s13256-015-0619-3.
18. Hudthagosol C, Haddad E, and R Jongsuwat. 2012. Antioxidant activity comparison of walnuts and fatty fish. *Journal of the Medical Association of Thailand*, Jun; 95(Suppl 6): S179–S188. PMID: 23130505.
19. Willcox DC, Scapagnini G, and BJ Willcox. 2014. Healthy aging diets other than the Mediterranean: a focus on the Okinawan diet. *Mechanisms of Ageing and Development*, Mar–Apr 2014; 136–137: 148–62. DOI: 10.1016/j.mad.2014.01.002.

3 Omegas Strengthen Your Blood Vessels and Your Heart

> Those who take medicine and neglect their diet waste the skill of the physician.
>
> —Chinese proverb

3.1 WHAT YOU DON'T KNOW SURELY WILL HURT YOU

Here's an all-too-common scene:

Doctor: I have your lab reports here, Charlie.
Patient: (Jokingly) Well, Doc, will I live?
Doctor: Of course, it's not that bad. But you will have to make some changes. You know that your blood pressure has been somewhat elevated for some time now and your cholesterol levels and triglycerides are also high.
Patient: What should I do?
Doctor: I will give you prescriptions to lower your blood pressure—this includes a diuretic—and to lower your cholesterol and you need to pay attention to your diet and lose some weight … and do more exercise.

This kind of advice is so common that it is clichéd. "You need to pay attention to your diet." Also common is, "Yes, you can drink in moderation … a glass or two of wine a day."

A glass or two of wine a day can lead to addiction and, besides, alcohol promotes the formation of Reactive Oxygen Species (ROS), those nasty ROS detailed in the last chapter. Alcohol metabolism results in formation of *acetaldehyde* that leads to liver impairment, for one thing, increasing the level of free iron that can turn to rust in your cells and reducing the levels of antioxidants such as glutathione (GSH). Bingo! Oxidative stress (1).

"Aw, jeez, just a glass or two, Doc?"

If left to his own devices, this typical patient will likely see his health worsen. Statistics from the Centers for Disease Control and Prevention (CDC) tell us that. He will most likely take his meds … more or less. Non-adherence to medication(s) is widely recognized as a common and costly problem. According to a 2005 report in the *New England Journal of Medicine*, approximately 30–50% of US adults are not compliant with long-term medications, leading to an estimated $100 billion in preventable costs annually (2).

Charlie will not lose weight. In fact, he will gain more, and he will be even more sedentary as he ages. He may develop essential (chronic) hypertension and atherosclerosis poorly controlled by prescription meds. He will drink more alcohol, and possibly, he may even be a smoker. He may progress to kidney failure and heart failure and graduate to a coronary heart attack. The CDC tells us that.

What could that doctor have told him instead of "watch your diet"? How about, "Charlie, you gotta skip the hamburgers and fries and get into eating flax muffins for breakfast, and some fish two or three times a week."

So, there are three health-related dreads that regularly haunt us Americans now: Cardiovascular disease, premature aging and shorter lifespan. Cancer runs a close fourth. And, what's worse, they are related. There's no getting away from it, they're out there. We read about them, we hear about them and we see it on TV. In fact, they are "the elephant in the room." Everything we contemplate eating, whatever exercise we plan to engage in, there's always an element of "But what if … or what if I don't. Does this cause …?"

These dreaded conditions are very common here. It is clear that they are somehow related to the fractured oxygen atoms we call free radicals that broke apart in metabolism or were caused by stuff like smog in the air we breathe; that these corrode our body when they combine with sugar, saturated fats or proteins in the body; and that what we eat can make it better or worse. But, other than to scare them, most Americans only know vaguely what they are.

First, the things that commonly ail us such as hypertension, atherosclerosis, coronary heart disease, Type 2 diabetes, metabolic syndrome and chronic kidney disease, arthritis … even glaucoma, are due to damage to a particular organ in the body that most people have probably never heard of—an organ most of our doctors likely did not know about until the 1980s. It wasn't even shown in most anatomical illustrations in their textbooks. Yet, it is the largest organ in the body; it is highly susceptible to damage by ROS, and when it is damaged, it jeopardizes everything else in the body. "What organ is that?" It is called the "endothelium."

The endothelium is shown in Figure 3.1. It is made up of a single layer of cells that form the inner lining of all of our blood vessels, i.e., arteries, arterioles, venules, veins and capillaries, even the lymph vessels.

The endothelial cells form that accordion-like fluted inner lining of all blood vessels and there's at least one trillion of those endothelial cells in each person. They would weigh in at more than 100 grams (g) and if one could stretch it out as a sheet, the endothelium would cover an area of about 3,000 square meters (m^2), that's almost 10,000 square feet (ft^2). That's ten times the size of a tennis court. Even your skin would only cover an area of about 22 ft^2.

Because the endothelium is fluted like an accordion, it makes it possible for it to expand and contract as blood vessels expand and constrict to change the volume of blood flow to accommodate changes in activity. Were it not fluted, it would tear apart the first time we ran, and we'd be done for.

What we don't see in the illustration is that there is an even smaller, gummy layer that lies over the endothelium in the vessel lumen. It cannot be seen at this magnification. It is called the glycocalyx. It is made up of various sugar/protein-like compounds and it protects the cells of the endothelium from the blood rushing past

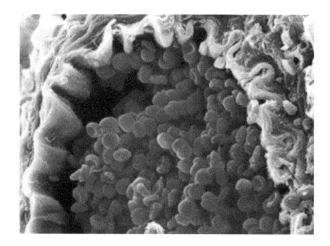

FIGURE 3.1 Colored scanning electron micrograph (SEM) of a cross-section through a small human arteriole. Red blood cells are seen in the central space (lumen) surrounded by the fluted endothelial cell lining that stretches enabling the arteriole to expand and contract. (From https://www.pinterest.co.uk/pin/448600812867071055/. With permission.)

them. It is also a barrier to excess salt, excess sugar, bacteria, viruses and of course ROS in the bloodstream. This is a vital protection, and it is vital that we protect it. And omega-3s will do just that for us.

By the way, Covid-19 can get us by attacking our blood vessels. It can damage them because it can get through the endothelium by damaging the glycocalyx barrier (3).

High blood pressure damages the endothelium. Atherosclerosis damages the endothelium. Type 2 diabetes damages the endothelium. ROS damage the endothelium. High blood sugar damages the glycocalyx exposing the endothelium to damage. High dietary sodium (salt is one form) damages the glycocalyx exposing the endothelium to damage. And those are the main but not the only threats to the endothelium. And an impaired endothelium causes *all* those cardiovascular diseases—no less coronary heart attacks from which almost 700,000 Americans died in 2020.

"Well so what?" is what the entire medical community said about the endothelium until now because no one knew, nor did anyone care what the endothelium did until the 1980s when that became the basis for a Nobel Prize in Medicine awarded to three American scientists, Robert F. Furchgott, Ferid Murad and Louis J. Ignarro in 1998.

The benefits of the omegas, 3 and 6, but especially high levels of the 3s, is that they can avert damage to and impairment of the endothelium and consequent catastrophe.

3.2 IT'S A GAS

In the early 1900s, the Austrian pharmacologist Otto Loewi discovered a substance made by nerve cells in the brain and in the body. Some years later, Sir Henry Dale, with whom Loewi later collaborated at the University of London, and with whom he shared the 1936 Nobel Prize in Medicine, named it "acetylcholine" (ACh). This was the beginning of the modern science of chemical signals called *neurotransmitters* by which cells in the nervous system and brain communicate and regulate activities.

Medicine had been searching for a "cure" for chronically elevated blood pressure since the 1940s—President Franklin D. Roosevelt died of its *untreated* complications—and ACh was found to relax the arterial blood vessels all throughout the circulatory system and this seemed a promising road to lower blood pressure to treat hypertension, except that it did so unreliably and unpredictably. No one knew why.

In 1980, Dr Robert F. Furchgott, professor of pharmacology at Downstate Medical Center in Brooklyn, NY, published his findings in the journal *Nature* that ACh relaxation of arterial blood vessels depended on the simultaneous presence of a mysterious substance actually made by the *endothelium*. The mysterious substance was initially termed *"endothelium-derived relaxing factor"* (EDRF) because ACh relaxed the blood vessels only when that factor was also present (4), but no one had any idea what it actually was.

Then, in 1993, Dr Salvador Moncada at Wellcome Research Labs, UK, first identified EDRF as a gas, nitric oxide (NO), and detailed its role in health and disease in the *New England Journal of Medicine* (NEJM) (5). NO is derived by the cells of the endothelium principally from the food-borne amino acid L-arginine found in proteins, and also from dietary nitrates such as green leafy vegetables, cruciferous vegetables, cabbage and especially beets. And at first, this news was met with disbelief—even derision. A gas, indeed! It was not known then that NO had a biological role, much less in blood vessels.

Then in 1998, Dr Furchgott and those two colleagues were awarded the Nobel Prize in Medicine for the discovery of the biological role of NO in blood vessels and heart function. This immediately propelled the endothelium into the medical limelight. Now it was finally understood that all those dreaded cardiovascular diseases were due to the failure of the endothelium to form NO, and NO controlled blood circulation throughout the body and the brain, and it controlled the function of the heart.

And then, one of the three recipients, Dr Ignarro, detailed how in sexual arousal, ACh led to increased and sustained production of NO by the endothelium lining the spongy chambers of the penis. This causes them to relax (dilate) allowing increased blood inflow and, thus, erection. He went on to devise a way to increase endothelial NO availability by administering a compound, calling it VIAGRA®.

It soon followed that the failure of the endothelium to form NO was discovered to be principally caused by ROS damage and that established the role of nutrition in its health and in disease. If you enter "how ROS damage endothelium" in PubMed (National Library of Medicine), you will be served with 25,647 medical science journal articles to choose from.

3.3 HOW A SIMPLE "BLUNDER" EXPLAINS CARDIOVASCULAR AND HEART DISEASE

When the body releases ACh into the bloodstream, it should invariably cause the formation of NO by the endothelium of arterial blood vessels, causing them to relax and increase blood flow. So why didn't it do that reliably in Dr Furchgott's laboratory?

What Dr Furchgott discovered when he immersed strips of arterial blood vessels in an ACh solution is that the strips did not relax when on closer examination it was found that laboratory preparation had actually damaged the endothelium—it had rubbed away a lot of cells. A simple blunder, perhaps? But it was soon learned that damaged endothelium can't form NO. And this turned out to be a very important lesson for medicine with far reaching implications for cardiovascular health.

The observation that damaged endothelium can't produce NO in amounts sufficient to cause blood vessel dilation and maintain adequate blood circulation is the explanation for how we come by cardiovascular disorders such as hypertension, atherosclerosis, heart failure, kidney disease and metabolic syndrome; and now we can add erectile dysfunction (ED) as well. Each of these conditions is said to result from damage to the endothelium—as sure as if it were "rubbed" away—and each, in turn, causes further damage to the endothelium.

But, in the population at risk, it is mostly diet and lifestyle factors favoring the formation of ROS—especially a low antioxidant diet—that damage the endothelium—that rub it away, as it were. Anyone with a high-fat, high-salt, high-sugar diet or hypertension and/or atherosclerosis, or Type 2 diabetes, is replicating the outcome of that laboratory blunder. To supply adequate oxygen and nutrients to all parts of our body, and to eliminate carbon dioxide and wastes, our endothelium must be healthy and able to form NO on demand when and where needed in the body.

In the following sections, we will first report the scientific evidence that many of the foods that we consume damage the endothelium by causing it to be pummeled with ROS, thus impairing its ability to form NO, and then we will show how antioxidant omega-3s can prevent, even restore and rejuvenate, damaged endothelium.

Bottom line: When you're out of NO, you're out of gas.

3.4 HOW DOES DIET DAMAGE THE ENDOTHELIUM?

There are many ways that the endothelium can be damaged. Endothelial dysfunction can result from bacterial or viral infection, atherosclerosis, hypertension, oxidative stress through inadequate antioxidant opposition of ROS, and so on. But the one for which we could be most responsible is our nutrition habits—the foods we consume … and those we don't consume.

The first stage in the development of atherosclerosis is endothelial dysfunction resulting in impairment of NO formation. Endothelial dysfunction is invariably present in people with cardiovascular disease and/or coronary risk factors, such as hypertension, elevated blood lipids, Type 2 diabetes and people with elevated blood levels of homocysteine (resulting from vitamin B-12 or folate deficiency). According to a report in 2010 in the *Journal of Cardiology*, smoking is a very effective way to damage the endothelium (6).

It has been shown that dietary factors may benefit endothelial function and thus blood vessel health. Nutrients, such as fish oil, antioxidants, L-arginine, folic acid and soy protein have resulted in improvement in endothelial function that reduces the risk of cardiovascular disease. There is some evidence suggesting that the Mediterranean Diet characterized by high consumption of vegetables, fish, olive oil and even "moderate" wine consumption may have a positive effect on endothelial function (7).

3.5 HEALTHY FOOD PATTERNS VS UNHEALTHY FOOD PATTERNS

We learn from a report published in 2014, in the *Journal of Clinical Hypertension*, about evidence for food patterns and markers of endothelial dysfunction. Healthy food patterns were those abundant in fruits and vegetables and they had a beneficial impact on endothelial function as estimated by circulating levels of inflammation biomarkers such as C-Reactive Protein (CRP). The level of CRP increases when there's inflammation in the body.

Westernized diet patterns with higher intakes of processed meats, sweets, fried foods and refined grains were significantly associated with inflammation and promoters of atherosclerosis (8).

3.5.1 High-Sodium Diet

We generally think of elevated blood pressure as the main harm done by a high dietary sodium intake, but that is only the tip of the iceberg. We learn from a report published in 2021 in the journal *Nutrients*, that despite decades of efforts to reduce sodium intake, excess dietary sodium is still very much commonplace, and that it contributes to increased risk of cardiovascular disease and death … and that is independent of the effects of excess sodium on blood pressure.

The authors of that study published in the journal *Nutrients*, in 2021, contend that high-sodium diets lead to impaired endothelial function and reduced NO availability even in the absence of a change in blood pressure (9). In fact, a high-salt diet damages the glycocalyx barrier protecting the endothelium from harmful substances and bacteria, and viruses, in the bloodstream. This leaves the endothelium also more vulnerable to ROS (10).

3.5.2 High-Animal Fat Diet

High-fat diets are associated with endothelial dysfunction. The aim of a 2015 study published in the journal *Applied Physiology, Nutrition and Metabolism* was to determine how dietary fat intake affects the way that the endothelium controls blood circulation. The participants were middle-aged and older, sedentary, healthy adults. Some consumed a lower-fat diet and others consumed a high-fat diet. Four-day diet records were used to assess fat intake, and classifications were based on the American Heart Association guidelines (less than 35% of total calories from fat).

It was found that a high-fat diet is associated with endothelium dysfunction due, in part, to diminished NO availability and the investigators concluded that this impairment may contribute to the increased cardiovascular risk with high dietary fat intake (11).

3.5.3 HIGH-CARBOHYDRATE DIET

High carbohydrate-induced elevated blood sugar causes ROS formation that impairs blood vessel function. A report in 2015, in the journal *Clinical Nutrition Research*, concludes that maintaining recommended carbohydrate intake with low glycemic index* foods results in a better functioning circulatory system (12).

One of the commonest causes of coronary heart attack in people with Type 2 diabetes is damage to the endothelium (13). Chronically elevated blood sugar, as well as blood sugar spikes, causes glucose-based ROS to erode the glycocalyx, damaging the endothelium to the point that it actually ruptures. Blood pressure, as previously noted, no matter how elevated, is simply not enough to rupture a blood vessel unless it is damaged ... by atherosclerosis, for instance, or by continuous exposure to unopposed ROS.

The example above shows how foods can be adverse or beneficial in their effects on the viability of the endothelium and that is essential to its ability to synthesize NO, the gas/neurotransmitter molecule that controls how blood vessels manage blood flow to all parts of the body. Many things can impair endothelium health, but omega-3 fatty acids (FAs) can prevent damage and even restore healthy function after damage has occurred.

Many studies support the beneficial effects of omega-3 FAs on endothelial function. In some instances, it is from flaxseed oil-derived alpha-linolenic acid (ALA) (14), and in others, it is eicosapentaenoic acid (EPA) + docosahexaenoic acid (DHA) typically from fish or fish oil (15). To keep blood flowing in the volume required by activity, blood vessels need to be able to relax and expand as necessary to meet the blood flow demanded by a given level of activity. In order to meet those needs, the endothelium must be able to form NO so that the vessel can relax, expand and increase blood flow volume.

Sadly, as shown above, we have many opportunities, mostly from our diet, to jeopardize endothelium NO formation. A diet high in salt, high in sugar and simple carbs, high in saturated fats and low in antioxidants will do just that. These damage the glycocalyx protecting the endothelium and they damage the endothelium directly as well ... mostly by firing frequent volleys of ROS at those structures.

Of course, endothelium-formed NO is not the only mechanism that controls blood flow volume in the circulatory system. There are also other *neurotransmitters* such as ACh, which dilates blood vessels and slows the heart rate, and norepinephrine (noradrenaline), which increases the heart rate and raises blood pressure. But NO is the only one that we can directly improve or damage by our nutrition and our behavior, i.e., the well-known "lifestyle factors."

Just as blood vessels have an endothelium lining, the heart has a similar structure and it is made of the same type of cells and it is called the *endocardium*, and it is

---

* The Glycemic Index (GI) is a value used to measure how much a given food raises blood sugar levels. Low glycemic index foods include vegetables such as peppers, broccoli, tomatoes, lettuce, eggplants; fruits including strawberries, apples, pears; legumes including chickpeas, beans; dairy including whole/full-fat milk, plain yogurt; sweets such as dark chocolate with more than 70% cocoa; and nuts, including cashews, walnuts and peanuts.

also under the control of NO. The heart falters, just as a car stalls, when we run out of the gas NO.

Now, everybody knows that the heart is the pump that keeps blood flowing throughout our body at a more or less constant rate and more or less constant pressure. Right? But here's a question for you:

Suppose you went into a garden/hardware supply store and asked the salesperson for a pump the size of your fist that can pump fluid with the density of maple syrup through 60,000 miles of flexible hose ranging in diameter from 2.5 centimeters (cm) (large artery) to 10 micrometers (μm) (capillary, ten millionths of a meter), at a pressure around 2.3 pounds (lbs)/square inch. Don't you think that the salesperson would think that you are joking? That salesperson would laugh at you: "Are you kidding? No pump the size of your fist could do that."

Well, the majority of medical doctors are convinced that it can do that—but the salesperson is actually right. What the heart actually does is to "eject" blood into your circulatory system. That's it. Your blood vessels then do the rest of the pumping. That vast system of blood vessels making up the pump depends on *compliance*, i.e., flexibility so it can expand on the upstroke, and compliance depends on NO. Compliance therefore stands or falls on the outcome of the battle of antioxidants with ROS and that's where omega-3s come in.

We will show you where omega-3s come in at every step of the process of pumping blood throughout your body, and you will see clearly why it falters into cardiovascular disease risk without them.

3.6 AT THE HEART OF THE MATTER

Systole: The normal heart (Figure 3.2 is a "cutaway" illustration) has two upper and two lower chambers. The upper chambers, the right and left atria, receive incoming blood, shown in blue. Blue typically indicates that there is less than normal oxygen (O_2) content, whereas red indicates properly oxygenated blood. In fact, the veins in the wrist appear blue because veins usually carry less oxygenated blood than arteries.

The lower chambers, the more muscular right and left ventricles, eject blood out of the heart. The heart valves, which keep blood flowing in the right direction, are gates at the entrance to the chambers, preventing blood flowing back after the ventricle chambers contract.

The bent red arrow in the left ventricle shows the direction in which blood moves. It comes from the left atrium into the left ventricle, then, when the heart contracts, i.e., systole, it moves past the aortic valve into the aorta, and from there into the circulatory system. After the heart contracts, i.e., systole, the aortic valve closes so that blood cannot flow back from the aorta into the heart.

The action of the left ventricle is of great concern because it can malfunction for various reasons, thus seriously affecting blood circulation. For instance, sustained hypertension can cause the left ventricle to enlarge. That is called hypertrophy. This ultimately weakens it, possibly leading to *congestive heart failure* where body fluid builds up due to poor heart function.

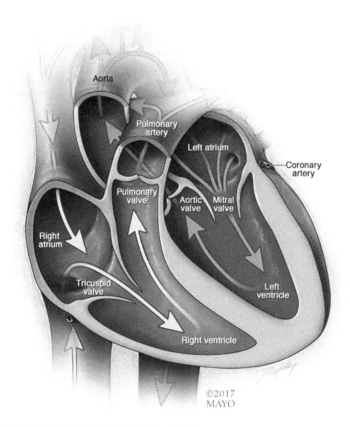

FIGURE 3.2 The four chambers of the heart and the direction of blood flow. (Used with permission of Mayo Foundation for Medical Education and research, all rights reserved.)

The adequacy of the pumping action of the heart is determined by what doctors call the "ejection fraction," that is the amount—percentage actually—of blood that is ejected, i.e., pumped out by each contraction of the ventricle as a glob of blood into the aorta and thus into the bloodstream.

But the left ventricle does not eject all the blood it contains with each contraction and so the efficiency of the heart is determined by the percentage of the blood it contains that is actually "ejected" into the blood circulation with each beat. A normal heart ejection fraction may be between 50% and 70%. Ejection fraction under 40% may be evidence of "heart failure."

Just as blood vessels have an endothelial lining that participates in the function of the vessel, so the heart has a parallel inner surface lining, the *endocardium*. The *endocardium* consists of a layer of endothelial cells and an underlying layer of connective tissue. Therefore, the action of the heart, just like that of arterial blood vessels, is regulated not only by the neurotransmitters ACh and norepinephrine, but to a great extent by the action of NO as well. And, just like blood vessels, its function is jeopardized by anything that impairs the availability of NO such as a damaged endocardium. ROS come to mind (16).

The adequacy of the pumping action of the heart also depends on the synchrony of the sequence of the chamber contractions. One study showed that one form of asynchrony (arrhythmia), the well-known and not so uncommon atrial fibrillation (AFib), disrupts the formation of NO by the endocardium. Apparently, atrial fibrillation reduces the ability of the endocardium to form NO as needed and this can also lead to stroke (17).

Blood flowing to the heart proper is delivered by the two-branch (right and left) coronary arteries encircling the surface of the heart. When the heart contracts, i.e., systole, the aortic valve opens as it ejects a portion of the contents of the left ventricle into the aorta. Then the valve closes. Understanding what happens next is the key to understanding why NO is crucial to blood circulation. But, exactly how dependent is heart function on NO availability?

According to a report in *Science Daily* (May 14, 2018), "Heart disease severity may depend on nitric oxide levels: study finds nitric oxide may also determine drug efficacy" (18). The report informs us that not only is NO deficiency a key feature of heart disease, but meds intended to treat it don't work well when NO is insufficiently available. The authors of the study on which the report is based state unequivocally that: "In addition, our results point to the possibility that heart failure may represent different clinical conditions depending on NO bioavailability" (19).

According to another report in the journal *Life Sciences*, titled "Nitric oxide and cardiac function," NO is a key element in the control of heart contraction (20). In fact, reduced NO bioavailability imposes an upper limit on blood flow regulation to the heart muscles proper and its transmission of blood throughout the heart (21).

Flaxseed omega-3 FA alpha-linolenic acid (ALA), is just what the doctor (should have) ordered. It promotes NO formation by the endocardium. But many investigators who tout omega-3 FAs for heart health seem unaware of the NO connection. For instance, in a study titled "The cardiovascular effects of flaxseed and its omega-3 fatty acid, alpha-linolenic acid," reported in the *Canadian Journal of Cardiology*, in 2010, we are told that preventing cardiovascular disease with nutritional interventions by increased use of omega-3 FAs may have significant cardiovascular benefits. The report proposes "marine" food FAs (22). But no mention is made of the role of the omega-3 in promoting endothelial health and NO formation.

Even the medical establishment does not get to hear about all this. So why then would it recommend diets that promote endothelium health and NO availability? It is up to us to learn how all this fits together and to implement an endothelium-saving nutrition plan. A number of them are detailed later in the book.

Many other studies have reported that flaxseed has recently gained attention in connection with reducing cardiovascular disease risk because it is the richest known source of both ALA and the phytoestrogen, lignans, as well as being a good source of soluble fiber (23). Lignans are phytoestrogens that effectively lower the risk of heart disease (24).

In patients with atherosclerosis, ejection fraction improves from 45% to 55% with flaxseed. A low ejection fraction, e.g., 45% or less, is evidence of heart failure. Flaxseed improves the ejection fraction. It was reported in the *Journal of Molecular and Cellular Cardiology* that patients with atherosclerosis showed improved ejection fraction—from 45% to 55% —when given an antioxidant phytoestrogen from flaxseed (25). One study, published in the journal *Nutrients* in 2017, went so far as to propose supplementing omega-3 FAs (from fish oil) based on their findings that it improved ejection fraction in heart failure patients (26). That recommendation is not widely implemented.

So far, we have shown that when the heart contracts, the left ventricle ejects a glob of blood into the aorta. If it can eject only a small fraction of the total volume of blood in that ventricle, there is the makings of heart failure. That failure is often ascribed to inadequate formation and availability of NO: NO is produced from virtually all cell types that make up heart muscle and regulate heart function (27).

But what happens *after* the ejection of a glob of blood—normal or subnormal—into the bloodstream ... and what've omega-3s got to do with it? The answer depends on "compliance," and if one does not have it, it's big trouble. And, if one has atherosclerosis and, therefore can't make enough NO, they haven't got it. Omega-3s can correct that fault.

3.7 ARTERIAL VESSEL COMPLIANCE

After systole, when the glob of blood is ejected from the left ventricle into the bloodstream, i.e., into the aorta, the large artery that leaves the heart, then becomes *diastole*. That's "where the rubber hits the road," as they say.

But the aorta is not empty. It still has some blood in it from the last contraction. And so the volume of the glob ejected into the aorta is added to the volume of blood that is still there after the last systole. Therefore, the vessel must momentarily distend—bulge outward quite a bit, as a matter of fact. Here is where it needs to be elastic, and compliance can be understood as elasticity.

That segment of the aorta needs to be able to stretch out to accommodate the new glob of blood and then to spring back to its original shape to push it forward. That, by the way is the actual pump—artery expansion/contraction, artery expansion/contraction and so on, all along the entire circulatory system (Figure 3.3).

If you look at the left part, A (elastic arteries), that is how normal blood vessels work. They distend and they spring back. But, in B (stiff arteries), abnormal arteries, they barely distend at all. They are not elastic. They do not "comply." That's what happens in atherosclerosis—hardening of the arteries—and that's why hypertension, i.e., chronic elevated blood pressure, usually goes hand in hand with it.

So, medicine usually warns us that hardening of the arteries can result in *ruptures* in plaques causing potentially fatal blood clots. True enough. But medicine never tells us about compliance, i.e., how the pump works and how we can damage it. So, even long before it gets to the point of rupture, impaired compliance raises the risk of heart attack.

It will not surprise you to know that the pump is powered by gas, as it were: Omega-3 FAs promote endocardium health and therefore NO formation.

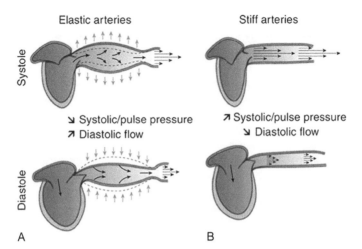

FIGURE 3.3 Schematic representation of the role of arterial compliance (i.e., the inverse of arterial stiffness) in assuring blood flow through the peripheral circulation. (From Briet, Boutouyrie, Laurent et al. 2012. *Kidney International* (28). With permission.)

3.8 FLAXSEED OIL PROMOTES ARTERIAL BLOOD VESSEL ELASTICITY (COMPLIANCE)

The risk of cardiovascular catastrophe rises with the decline in the compliance or elasticity of arterial blood vessels. Conversely, arterial compliance improves when one consumes foods that supply omega-3 FAs.

When people with insulin resistance were given an *alpha*-linolenic acid/low fat regimen, their blood vessel compliance rose significantly. In a study, published in 1997 in the journal *Arteriosclerosis, Thrombosis, and Vascular Biology*, it was reported that when obese people with markers for insulin resistance ate, in turn, four separate diets of 4 weeks duration each: saturated/high fat (SHF), alpha-linolenic acid/low fat (ALF), oleic/low fat (OLF) and then SHF again. Daily intake of ALA was 20 g from margarine products based on flax oil. Arterial compliance was calculated from aortic blood flow velocity and pressure. Plasma lipids, glucose tolerance and in vitro low density lipoprotein (LDL) oxidizability were also measured.

It was found that blood vessel compliance rose significantly with the *alpha*-linolenic acid/low fat (ALF) regimen. Insulin sensitivity increased significantly. The investigators concluded that dietary omega-3 FAs improve arterial blood vessel function (29).

There's a simple way to see if one has "compliance." Here's a little-known trick: If one doesn't already have a pulse oximeter that shows pulse waveform, they can get one online or at a pharmacy. For instance, the Innovo Deluxe iP900AP Fingertip Pulse Oximeter with Plethysmograph and Perfusion Index can be purchased for $34.00 on *Amazon*. Many other similar units can be found for sale on the internet.

The first part of the waveform rises with systole as the blood glob is ejected into the aorta. Then the valve between the heart and the aorta closes so that blood cannot flow backwards into the heart. That is diastole. In that phase, the vessel having complied, it springs back, and the glob is pushed forward into the bloodstream. Without going further into it, the notch in the descending part of the waveform is called the *dicrotic notch*. It is present in elastic arteries that have compliance (30). It is very shallow or missing in stiff arteries.

Daily omega-3 supplementation decreases arterial stiffness in older adults. In other words, it increases arterial compliance. The journal *Physiological Reports* published a clinical study in 2015 titled "Effect of omega-3 polyunsaturated fatty acid supplementation on central arterial stiffness and arterial wave reflections in young and older healthy adults." Based on changes in pulse waveform, the authors concluded that 12 weeks of daily omega-3 supplementation decreases central arterial stiffness in older adults (31). Just 3 months of consuming foods or supplements rich in omega-3 FAs can bring about a major reduction in arterial stiffness and thus reduce the risk of cardiovascular disorders that are commonly fatal.

3.9 OMEGA-3s "LUBRICATE" YOUR HEART VALVES

You can see in Figure 3.2, the cutaway illustration of the heart, that there are four valves which open and close with each heartbeat. Blood has to flow in just one direction, and they close to prevent it from flowing backwards during a pause (diastole). Then, when the heart contracts they open again as blood flows forward. Diseased valves can become "leaky" where they don't completely close causing what is called "regurgitation." If this happens, blood leaks back into the chamber that it came from, and not enough blood can be pushed forward through the heart. Or the valves can become stiff, inflexible.

According to the CDC, about 2.5% of the US population has heart valve disease, but it is more common in older adults. About 13% of people born before 1943 are affected. In 2017, 61% of deaths due to valve disease were due to aortic valve *stenosis*, a thickening and narrowing of the valve. That narrowing creates a smaller opening for blood to pass through, reducing or blocking blood flow from the heart to the rest of the body.

Omega-3 FAs slow the progression of aortic valve disease. In 2020, *Circulation*, the journal of the American Heart Association, published a clinical study titled "Omega-3 polyunsaturated fatty acids decrease aortic valve disease." In their report, the investigators describe aortic valve stenosis, the most common valvular heart disease, as a progressive narrowing of the aortic valve due to thickening of and calcium accumulation on the valve leaflets. Based on previous findings of the beneficial effects of omega-3 FAs in cardiovascular disease prevention, they aimed to see if omega-3 FAs could be of benefit in aortic valve stenosis.

It was found that omega-3 FAs inhibited the progression of aortic valve stenosis, and the investigators recommended it as a "novel potential therapeutic opportunity to be evaluated in patients with AVS" (32).

3.10 OMEGA-3s PROTECT THE CORONARY ARTERIES

We hear much about the killer "coronary heart disease," AKA coronary artery disease. No wonder. It is a type of heart disease that develops when the arteries of the heart cannot deliver enough oxygen-rich blood to the heart, and it is the leading cause of death in the United States. There's actually a number of different forms but most often it is caused by the buildup of atherosclerotic plaque inside the walls of larger coronary arteries. This buildup can partially or totally block blood flow, thus suffocating regions of the heart. In certain circumstances, it can even result in a rupture in the coronary artery.

Regularly consuming omega-3 FAs from marine sources and plant sources prevents cardiac death as well as nonfatal heart attacks. In 2001, the journal *Archives of Internal Medicine* published a report aptly titled "The fats of life." The authors tell us that there is good reason to believe that omega-3 FAs can prevent coronary heart disease: Dietary sources of omega-3 FAs include fish oils rich in EPA and DHA, as well as plants rich in ALA.

According to the authors, fish oils reduce the risk of heart "events" with an efficacy equal to that seen in secondary prevention trials with lipid-lowering drugs. Secondary prevention includes regular exams and screening tests to detect disease in its earliest stages (e.g., mammograms to detect breast cancer); daily, low-dose aspirin and/or diet and exercise programs to prevent further heart attacks or strokes. It is thought that risk reduction is due to prevention of heart arrhythmias, to lowering of blood lipids and to reducing the risk of blood clots—all said to be due to consuming fish oil.

The authors tell us that fish is an important source of omega-3 FAs in the US diet, but that vegetable sources, including grains and oils, are an alternative source for those who can't consume fish regularly. They summarize evidence from published clinical studies on patients with coronary heart disease that show that intake of omega-3 FAs from marine sources and/or plant sources prevent cardiac death as well as nonfatal heart attacks (33).

Regularly consuming fatty fish significantly lowers the risk of acute coronary syndrome in men. And a Danish study published in 2010, in the *European Heart Journal*, aimed to determine the effects of fish consumption on the risk of "acute coronary syndrome" (ACS) in healthy people. ACS describes conditions associated with sudden, reduced blood flow to the heart. It typically results in a heart attack and myocardial infarction, when heart cell death results in damaged or destroyed heart tissue.

The follow-up study included nearly 60,000 men and women between 50 and 64 years old. Intake of lean and fatty fish was estimated from a detailed and validated food frequency questionnaire. It was found that intake of fatty fish was associated with a significantly lower risk of acute coronary syndrome in men. The investigators concluded that a modest intake of fatty fish was associated with a lower risk of acute coronary syndrome (34).

This chapter began with that little fanciful scenario between the doctor and the patient that is all too common. One can only wonder why it is not more common that patients be given specific instructions about preventing or treating cardiovascular disease with both omega-3 and omega-6 FAs—in the proper ratio. After all, there is a considerable number of scientific reports that propose that, and we have shown but a small sample of them.

It is not likely that the physician who does not inform patients about this form of prevention and treatment simply does not know about it. Even the very conservative American Heart Association recommends omega-3s—and, curiously, they recommend *against* using multivitamin or mineral supplements to prevent cardiovascular diseases—curiously, because they're antioxidants. Here is what it says on their website:

Do this:

- Eat a healthy diet. There's just no substitute for a balanced, nutritious diet that limits excess calories, saturated fat, trans fat, sodium and dietary cholesterol. This approach has been shown to reduce coronary heart disease risk in healthy people and those with heart disease.
- Patients with heart disease should consume about 1 gram of omega-3 fatty acids called EPA + DHA. This should ideally come from fish.[*] This can be hard to get by diet alone, so a supplement could be needed. As always, consult with a physician first.
- If you have elevated triglycerides, try to get 2 to 4 grams per day of EPA+DHA.

Don't do this:

- Don't take antioxidant vitamin supplements such as A, C and E. Scientific evidence does not suggest these can eliminate the need to reduce blood pressure, lower blood cholesterol or stop smoking.
- Do not rely only on supplements. There isn't sufficient data to suggest that healthy people benefit by taking certain vitamin or mineral supplements in excess of the daily recommended allowance. Some observational studies have suggested that using these can lower rates of cardiovascular disease and/or lower risk factor levels.

> (https://www.heart.org/en/healthy-living/healthy-eating/eat-mart/ nutrition- basics/vitamin-supplements-hype-or-help-for-healthy- eating; accessed January 27, 2022)

They are opposed to antioxidants. And yet they propose taking omega-3 FA ... which are antioxidants.

Reading about how omega-3 FAs can lower and even prevent the risk of coming down with one of these dreadful diseases, it may become clear that it may not be so much a matter of what needs to be taken out of our diet, but a matter of what must be added to it—flax and fish mostly.

---

[*] It would also be helpful to tell people that Type 2 diabetes is common in people with heart disease and that fish can be high in iodine, and therefore can significantly raise blood sugar (35). Iodine has a half-life of 66.1 ± 6.3 days in normal persons; 38.2 ± 8.6 days in hyperthyroid persons; and 29.3 ± 8.8 days in hypothyroid persons (36).

3.11 OMEGA-3 FATTY ACIDS AND CARDIOVASCULAR DISEASE: NEW RECOMMENDATIONS FROM THE AMERICAN HEART ASSOCIATION (2003)

In 2003, the journal *Arteriosclerosis, Thrombosis, and Vascular Biology* published a comprehensive report titled "Omega-3 fatty acids and cardiovascular disease: new recommendations from the American Heart Association." The panel reported that people at risk for coronary heart disease could benefit from consuming omega-3 FAs from plants and marine sources. Studies cited recommended intakes of EPA + DHA ranging from 0.5 to 1.8 g per day (either as fatty fish or supplements) to significantly reduce the deaths from heart disease and all causes. These data support the Year 2000 AHA Dietary Guidelines recommendation to include at least two servings of fish (particularly fatty fish) per week. For ALA, a total intake of 1.5–3 g per day seems to be beneficial.

In patients with coronary heart disease, it was reported that omega-3 FA supplements significantly reduced death, nonfatal heart attacks and nonfatal strokes. What's more, omega-3 supplements can also slow the progression of atherosclerosis in these patients. Therefore, the American Heart Association (AHA) recommended that all adults eat fish (particularly fatty fish) at least two times a week. Fish, especially oily species like mackerel, lake trout, herring, sardines, albacore tuna and salmon, provide significant amounts of the two kinds of omega-3 FAs shown to be cardioprotective, EPA and DHA. The AHA also recommends eating plant-derived omega-3 FAs.

In addition, patients with documented coronary heart disease should consume approximately 1 g of EPA and DHA (combined) per day. This can be had in oily fish or from omega-3 FA capsules. The amount of EPA and DHA in fish and fish oil is presented in the recent AHA Scientific Advisory on omega-3 FAs and cardiovascular disease. Their table "Amounts of EPA + DHA in Fish and Fish Oils and the Amount of Fish Consumption Required to Provide ≈1 g of EPA + DHA per Day" can be accessed at https://www.ahajournals.org/doi/full/10.1161/01.CIR.0000038493.65177.94. It lists "EPA + DHA Content, g/3-oz Serving Fish (Edible Portion) or g/g Oil" and the "Amount Required to Provide ≈1 g of EPA + DHA per Day, oz (Fish) or g (Oil)."

The Omega-3 Fatty Acids Fact Sheet for Health Professionals on the National Institutes of Health, Office of Dietary Supplements website provides a table with omega-3 guidelines (Table 3.1).

We are also told that 2–4 g of EPA + DHA per day can lower triglycerides by 20–40%. However, patients taking more than 3 g of these FAs from supplements would be well advised to do so only under a physician's supervision.

The report also invokes a number of cautions:

- Very high intakes could cause excessive bleeding in some people.
- Some types of fish may contain significant levels of methylmercury, polychlorinated biphenyls (PCBs), dioxins and other environmental contaminants,[*] which are found predominantly in older, larger, predatory fish and marine mammals.

---

[*] Contaminants in fish and how to avoid them are reported in Chapter 8.

TABLE 3.1
ALA, EPA and DHA Content of Selected Foods

Food	Grams per Serving		
	ALA	DHA	EPA
Flaxseed oil, 1 tablespoon (tbsp)	7.26		
Chia seeds, 1 ounce (oz)	5.06		
English walnuts, 1 oz	2.57		
Flaxseed, whole, 1 tbsp	2.35		
Salmon, Atlantic, farmed cooked, 3 oz		1.24	0.59
Salmon, Atlantic, wild, cooked, 3 oz		1.22	0.35
Herring, Atlantic, cooked, 3 oz*		0.94	0.77
Canola oil, 1 tbsp	1.28		
Sardines, canned in tomato sauce, drained, 3 oz*		0.74	0.45
Mackerel, Atlantic, cooked, 3 oz*		0.59	0.43
Salmon, pink, canned, drained, 3 oz*	0.04	0.63	0.28
Soybean oil, 1 tbsp	0.92		
Trout, rainbow, wild, cooked, 3 oz		0.44	0.40
Black walnuts, 1 oz	0.76		
Mayonnaise, 1 tbsp	0.74		
Oysters, Eastern, wild, cooked, 3 oz	0.14	0.23	0.30
Sea bass, cooked, 3 oz*		0.47	0.18
Edamame, frozen, prepared, ½ cup	0.28		
Shrimp, cooked, 3 oz*		0.12	0.12
Refried beans, canned, vegetarian, ½ cup	0.21		
Lobster, cooked, 3 oz*	0.04	0.07	0.10
Tuna, light, canned in water, drained, 3 oz*		0.17	0.02
Tilapia, cooked, 3 oz*	0.04	0.11	
Scallops, cooked, 3 oz*		0.09	0.06
Cod, Pacific, cooked, 3 oz*		0.10	0.04
Tuna, yellowfin, cooked 3 oz*		0.09	0.01
Kidney beans, canned ½ cup	0.10		
Baked beans, canned, vegetarian, ½ cup	0.07		
Ground beef, 85% lean, cooked, 3 oz**	0.04		
Bread, whole wheat, 1 slice	0.04		
Egg, cooked, 1 egg		0.03	
Chicken, breast, roasted, 3 oz		0.02	0.01
Milk, low-fat (1%), 1 cup	0.01		

*   Except as noted, the USDA database does not specify whether fish are farmed or wild caught.
** The USDA database does not specify whether beef is grass fed or grain fed.
Source: https://ods.od.nih.gov/factsheets/Omega3FattyAcids-HealthProfessional/; accessed January 27, 2022.

Finally, the authors of the above-referenced study conclude that omega-3 FAs can significantly reduce the occurrence of unfortunate events in patients with coronary artery disease, based on the evidence from studies in which marine-derived omega-3 FAs have been consumed as fish or as supplements (37). Parenthetically, the second author of that publication, W.S. Harris, is the co-developer of the Omega-3 Index.

REFERENCES

1. Wu D, and AI Cederbaum. 2003. Alcohol, oxidative stress, and free radical damage. *Alcohol Research and Health*, 27(4): 277–284. PMID: 15540798.
2. Osterberg L, and T Blaschke. 2005. Adherence to medication. *New England Journal of Medicine*, Aug 4; 353(5):487–497. DOI: 10.1056/NEJMra050100.
3. Yamaoka-Tojo M. 2020. Vascular endothelial glycocalyx damage in COVID-19. *International Journal of Molecular Sciences*, Dec 19; 21(24): 9712. DOI: 10.3390/ijms21249712.
4. Furchgott RF, and JV Zawadzki. 1980. The obligatory role of endothelial cells in the relaxation of arterial smooth muscle by acetylcholine. *Nature*, Nov 27; 288(5789): 373–376. DOI: 10.1038/288373a0.
5. Moncada S, and A Higgs. 1993. The L-arginine-nitric oxide pathway. *New England Journal of Medicine*, Dec 30; 329(27):2002–2012. DOI: 10.1056/NEJM199312303292706.
6. Ozaki K, Hori T, Ishibashi T, Nishio M, and Y Aizawa. 2010. Effects of chronic cigarette smoking on endothelial function in young men. *Journal of Cardiology*, Nov; 56(3): 307–313. DOI: 10.1016/j.jjcc.2010.07.003.
7. Cuevas AM, and AM Germain. 2004. Diet and endothelial function. *Biological Research*, 37(2): 225–230. DOI: 10.4067/s0716-97602004000200008.
8. Defagó MD, Elorriaga N, Irazola VE, and AL Rubinstein. 2014. Influence of food patterns on endothelial biomarkers: A systematic review. *Journal of Clinical Hypertension (Greenwich)*, Dec; 16(12): 907–913. DOI: 10.1111/jch.12431.
9. Patik JC, Lennon SL, Farquhar WB, and DG Edwards. 2021. Mechanisms of dietary sodium-induced impairments in endothelial function and potential countermeasures. *Nutrients*. Jan; 13(1): 270. DOI: 10.3390/nu13010270.
10. Oberleithner H, Peters W, Kusche-Vihrog K, Korte S, Schillers H, Kliche K, and K Oberleithner. 2011. Salt overload damages the glycocalyx sodium barrier of vascular endothelium. *Pflugers Archives*, 462(4): 519–528. DOI: 10.1007/s00424-011-0999-1.
11. Dow CA, Stauffer BL, Greiner JJ, and CA DeSouz. 2015. Influence of habitual high dietary fat intake on endothelium-dependent vasodilation. *Applied Physiology, Nutrition and Metabolism*, Jul; 40(7): 711–715. DOI: 10.1139/apnm-2015-0006.
12. Jovanovski E, Zurbau A, and V Vuksan. 2015. Carbohydrates and endothelial function: Is a low-carbohydrate diet or a low glycemic index diet favourable for vascular health? *Clinical Nutrition Research*, Apr; 4(2): 69–75. DOI: 10.7762/ cnr.2015.4.2.69.
13. Dogné S, Flamion B, and Nathalie Caron. 2018. Endothelial glycocalyx as a shield against diabetic vascular complications. Involvement of hyaluronan and hyaluronidases. *Arteriosclerosis, Thrombosis and Vascular Biology*, Jul; 38(7): 1427–1439. DOI: 10.1161/ATVBAHA.118.310839.
14. Parikh M, Netticadan T, and GN Pierce. 2018. Flaxseed: its bioactive components and their cardiovascular benefits. *Heart and Circulatory Physiology*, 314: H146–H159. DOI:10.1152/ajpheart.00400.2017.

15. Zehr KR, and MK Walker. 2018. Omega-3 polyunsaturated fatty acids improve endothelial function in humans at risk for atherosclerosis: A review. *Prostaglandins and Other Lipid Mediators*, Jan; 134: 131–140. DOI: 10.1016/j prostaglandins. 2017.07.005.
16. Kellym RA, Balligand J-L, and TW Smith. 1996. Nitric oxide and cardiac function. *Circulation Research*, Sep; 79(3): 363–380. https://doi.org/10.1161/01.RES. 79.3.363.
17. Cai H, Li Z, Goette A, Mera F, Honeycutt C, Feterik K, Wilcox JN, Dudley SC, Harrison DG, and JJ Langberg. 2002. Downregulation of endocardial nitric oxide synthase expression and nitric oxide production in atrial fibrillation: Potential mechanisms for atrial thrombosis and stroke. *Circulation*, Nov; 106(22): 2854–2858.
18. www.sciencedaily.com/releases/2018/05/180514132501.htm; accessed 1/25/2.
19. Hayashi H, Hess DT, Zhang R, Sugi K, Gao H, Tan BL, Bowles DE, Milano CA, Jain MK, Koch WJ, and JS Stamler. 2018. S-Nitrosylation of β-Arrestins biases receptor signaling and confers ligand independence. *Molecular Cell*, May 3; 70(3): 473–487. DOI: 10.1016/j.molcel.2018.03.034.
20. Rastaldo R, Pagliaro P, Cappello S, Penna C, Mancardi D, Westerhof N, and G Losano. 2007. Nitric oxide and cardiac function. *Life Sciences*, Aug 16; 81(10): 779–793. DOI: 10.1016/j.lfs.2007.07.019.
21. Kingma Jr JG, Simard D, and JR Rouleau. 2015. Nitric oxide bioavailability affects cardiovascular regulation dependent on cardiac nerve status. *Autonomic Neuroscience*, Jan; 187: 70–75. DOI: 10.1016/j.autneu.2014.11.003.
22. Rodriguez-Leyva D, Bassett CMC, McCullough R, and GN Pierce. 2010. The cardiovascular effects of flaxseed and its omega-3 fatty acid, alpha-linolenic acid. *Canadian Journal of Cardiology*, Nov; 26(9): 489–496. DOI: 10.1016/s0828-282x(10)70455-4.
23. Bloedon LeAT, and PO Szapary. 2004. Flaxseed and cardiovascular risk. *Nutrition Reviews*, Jan; 62(1): 18–27. DOI: 10.1111/j.1753-4887.2004.tb00002.x.
24. Rodríguez-García C, Sánchez-Quesada C, Toledo E, Delgado-Rodríguez M, and JJ Gaforio. 2019. Naturally lignan-rich foods: A dietary tool for health promotion? *Molecules*, Mar; 24(5): 917. DOI: 10.3390/molecules24050917.
25. Penumathsa SV, Koneru S, Zhan L, John S, Menon VP, Prasad K, and N Maulik. 2008. Secoisolariciresinol diglucoside induces neovascularization-mediated cardioprotection against ischemia-reperfusion injury in hypercholesterolemic myocardium. *Journal of Molecular and Cellular Cardiology*, 44: 170–179. DOI: 10.1016/j.yjmcc.2007.09.014.
26. Wang C, Xiong B, and J Huang. 2017. The role of omega-3 polyunsaturated fatty acids in heart failure: A meta-analysis of randomised controlled trials. *Nutrients*, Jan; 9(1): 18. DOI: 10.3390/nu901001.
27. Massion PB, Feron O, Dessy C, and JL Balligand. 2003. Nitric oxide and cardiac function. Ten years after, and continuing. *Circulation Research*, 93(5): 388–398. https://doi.org/10.1161/01.RES.0000088351.58510.21.
28. Briet M, Boutouyrie P, Laurent S, and GM London. 2012. Arterial stiffness and pulse pressure in CKD and ESRD. *Kidney International*, Aug; 82(4): 388–400. DOI: 10.1038/ki.2012.131.
29. Nestel PJ, Pomeroy SE, Sasahara T, Yamashita T, Liang YL, Dart AM, Jennings JL, Abbey M, and JD Cameron.1997. Arterial compliance in obese subjects is improved with dietary plant n-3 fatty acid from flaxseed oil despite increased LDL oxidizability. *Arteriosclerosis, Thrombosis, and Vascular Biology*, Jun; 17(6): 1163–1170. DOI: 10.1161/01.atv.17.6.1163.
30. Rietzschel ER, and JA Chirinos. 2020. How to measure arterial stiffness in humans. *Arteriosclerosis, Thrombosis, and Vascular Biology*, 40: 1034–1043. https://doi.org/10.1161/ATVBAHA.119.313132.

31. Monahan KD, Feehan RP, Blaha C, and DJ McLaughlin. 2015. Effect of omega-3 polyunsaturated fatty acid supplementation on central arterial stiffness and arterial wave reflections in young and older healthy adults. *Physiological Reports*, Jun; 3(6): e12438. DOI: 10.14814/phy2.12438.
32. Artiach G, Carracedo M, Plunde O, Wheelock CE, Thul S, Sjövall P, Franco-Cereceda A, Laguna-Fernandez A, Arnardottir H, and M Bäck. 2020. Omega-3 polyunsaturated fatty acids decrease aortic valve disease through the Resolvin E1 and ChemR23 axis. *Circulation*, 142(8): 776–789. https://doi.org/10.1161/CIRCULA TIONAHA. 119.041868.
33. Harper CR, and TA Jacobson. 2001. The fats or life. *Archives of Internal Medicine*, 161(18): 2185–2192. DOI:10.1001/archinte.161.18.2185.
34. Bjerregaard LJ, Joensen AM, Dethlefsen C, Jensen MK, Johnsen SP, Tjønneland A, Rasmussen LH, Overvad K, and EB Schmidt. 2010. Fish intake and acute coronary syndrome. *European Heart Journal*, Jan; 31(1): 29–34. DOI: 10.1093/eurheartj/ ehp375.
35. Liu J, Liu L, Ji Q, Zhang X, Jin X, and H Shen. 2019. Effects of excessive iodine intake on blood glucose, blood pressure, and blood lipids in adults. *Biological Trace Elements Research*, Dec; 192(2): 136–144. DOI: 10.1007/s12011-019-01668-9.
36. Kramer GH. 2009. Retention of iodine in the body. In Preedy VR, Burrow GN, and R Watson, eds. *Comprehensive Handbook of Iodine*. Academic Press/Elsevier.
37. Kris-Etherton PM, Harris WS, Appel LJ, and the AHA Nutrition Committee. 2003. Omega-3 fatty acids and cardiovascular disease. New recommendations from the American Heart Association. *Arteriosclerosis, Thrombosis, and Vascular Biology*, 23(2): 151–152. https://doi.org/10.1161/01.ATV.0000057393.97337.AE.

4 Omega-3s and Hypertension, Atherosclerosis and Type 2 Diabetes

It is ambition enough to be employed as an under-labourer in clearing the ground a little, and removing some of the rubbish which lies in the way to knowledge.

—John Locke

4.1 ESSENTIAL HYPERTENSION

Blood pressure measurements were first performed in 1773 by Stephen Hales, a British clergyman. It was done on a horse by inserting a glass tube into a clamped artery. When the artery was untied, blood rose in the glass tube.

Essential hypertension, aka primary hypertension, is a medical term that boils down to chronic elevated blood pressure not due to a known medical condition. It is the most common type of hypertension, affecting about 85% of people with elevated blood pressure.

Normal blood pressure (bp) is said to be less than 120 millimeters of mercury (mm Hg) systolic and less than 80 mm Hg diastolic. When a blood pressure cuff has been inflated fully enough to occlude flow in the given artery, and the valve is then opened to start releasing pressure, the systolic pressure is the one that corresponds to either the first sound that one hears if using a stethoscope, or the first number to appear on the screen of a digital device. As the cuff continues to deflate, the diastolic pressure is either the last sound that one hears before it goes silent, or the second number to appear on the screen of a digital device. Millimeters of mercury is the conventional way to measure blood pressure. If one's blood pressure is not normal, they may be said to have:

- Prehypertension (mild): If systolic bp is between 120 and 139 mm Hg, or a diastolic bp between 80 and 89 mm Hg.
- Stage 1 (moderate): If systolic bp is between 140 and 159 mm Hg, or diastolic bp 90 and 99 mm Hg.
- Stage 2 (severe): If systolic bp is 160 mm Hg or higher, or diastolic bp is 100 mm Hg or higher, is hypertension.

4.2 WHAT ARE THE DANGERS OF HIGH BLOOD PRESSURE?

One can live for quite some time with elevated blood pressure without knowing it. In fact, most people with hypertension do exactly that. Do you remember the well-known admonition, "Don't get so aggravated ... watch your blood pressure or you'll get a stroke." Well, fortunately you can rest assured that if your blood vessels are reasonably healthy, you can't actually do that. Here's why:

Normal systolic blood pressure is, let's say, 120 mm Hg on average. That's 2.32 pounds (lbs) of pressure per square inch (psi). Normal diastolic blood pressure, when the heart is at rest between beats, is about 80 mm Hg. This translates to 1.55 psi. These are the pressure that blood exerts on the inner walls of blood vessels during the heartbeat cycle.

Suppose that for whatever reason, systolic blood pressure was grossly elevated to 220 mm Hg. That's 4.25 psi. You'll admit that's pretty high. But our brain capillaries have been shown to rupture and cause stroke only at an average pressure of 32.47 psi (1). That's more than seven times the 4.25 psi of a 220 mm Hg reading. To get to possible stroke pressure level, one would need a systolic blood pressure of about 1,679 mm Hg. Of course, this applies only to reasonably healthy blood vessels and that means an intact glycocalyx, a healthy endothelium and plaque-free and sludge-free blood vessel walls.

Now, if one has been subjecting their glycocalyx to a high-salt, high-sugar diet and liberally sprinkling viruses on it, engorging the blood vessel walls with atherosclerotic plaque, and targeting the endothelium with a barrage of Reactive Oxygen Species (ROS), all bets are off. And that's the whole point—only reasonably healthy blood vessels can take a lot of hits.

According to the Mayo Clinic, some people have high blood pressure caused by an underlying condition. This type of high blood pressure is called secondary hypertension, and it tends to appear suddenly and cause higher blood pressure than does primary hypertension. Various conditions and medications can lead to secondary hypertension, including:

- Obstructive sleep apnea.
- Kidney disease.
- Adrenal gland tumors.
- Thyroid problems.
- Certain defects in blood vessels one is born with (congenital).
- Certain medications, such as birth control pills, cold remedies, decongestants, over-the-counter pain relievers and some prescription drugs.
- Illegal drugs, such as cocaine and amphetamines.

High blood pressure entails many risk factors, including:

- *Age*. The risk of high blood pressure increases with age. Until about age 64, high blood pressure is more common in men. Women are more likely to develop high blood pressure after age 65.

- *Race.* High blood pressure is particularly common among people of African heritage, often developing at an earlier age than it does in white people.[*]
- *Family history.* High blood pressure tends to run in families.
- *Being overweight or obese.* The more one weighs, the more blood needed to supply oxygen and nutrients to body tissues. As the volume of blood flowing through the blood vessels increases, so does the pressure on artery walls.
- *Not being physically active.* People who are inactive tend to have higher heart rates. The higher the heart rate, the harder the heart must work with each contraction and the stronger the force exerted on the arteries.
- *Using tobacco.* Not only does smoking or chewing tobacco immediately raise blood pressure temporarily, but the chemicals in tobacco can damage the endothelium lining artery walls. Secondhand smoke also can increase the risk of heart disease.
- *Too much salt (sodium) in the diet.* Too much sodium in diet can cause the body to retain fluid, which increases blood pressure.
- *Too little potassium in the diet.* Potassium helps balance the amount of sodium in our cells. If you don't get enough potassium in the diet, or you lose too much potassium due to dehydration or other health conditions, sodium can build up in blood.
- *Drinking too much alcohol.* Over time, heavy drinking can damage the heart. Having more than one drink a day for women and more than two drinks a day for men may affect blood pressure. If one drinks alcohol, one is cautioned to do so in moderation. For healthy adults, that means up to one drink a day for women and two drinks a day for men.[†] One drink equals 12 ounces (oz) of beer, 5 oz of wine or 1.5 oz of 80-proof liquor.
- *Stress.* High levels of stress can lead to a temporary increase in blood pressure.
- *Certain chronic conditions.* Certain chronic conditions also may increase the risk of high blood pressure. This includes kidney disease, diabetes and sleep apnea.

Uncontrolled high blood pressure can lead to complications, including:

- *Heart attack or stroke.* High blood pressure can cause hardening and thickening of the arteries (atherosclerosis), which can lead to a heart attack, stroke or other complications.
- *Aneurysm.* Increased blood pressure can cause a blood vessel to bulge and weaken forming an aneurysm. If an aneurysm ruptures, it can be life-threatening.

---

[*] African Americans suffer from cardiovascular diseases at a rate about five times higher than the rest of the US population. According to a report published in the journal *Circulation* in 2004, many African Americans may develop a serious deficiency of nitric oxide (NO) formation resulting instead in the increased formation of a powerful ROS, peroxynitrite, enhancing oxidative stress (2).
[†] These are recommendations of the Mayo Clinic. We do not endorse anything other than an "occasional" drink. For one thing, alcohol is addictive. There are safer natural medicines.

- *Heart failure.* To pump blood against the higher pressure in our vessels, the heart has to work harder. This causes the walls of the heart pumping chamber to thicken (left ventricular hypertrophy). Eventually, the thickened muscle may have difficulty pumping enough blood to meet our body needs, and that can lead to heart failure.
- *Weakened and narrowed blood vessels in the kidneys.* This can prevent the kidneys from functioning normally.
- *Thickened, narrowed or torn blood vessels in the eyes.* This can result in loss of vision.
- *Metabolic syndrome.* This syndrome is a group of disorders of our body metabolism, including increased waist size, high triglycerides, decreased high-density lipoprotein (HDL) cholesterol (the "good" cholesterol), high blood pressure and high insulin levels. These conditions make you more likely to develop Type 2 diabetes, heart disease and stroke.
- *Trouble with memory or understanding.* Uncontrolled high blood pressure may also affect our ability to think, remember and learn. Trouble with memory or understanding concepts is more common in people with high blood pressure.
- *Dementia.* Narrowed or blocked arteries can limit blood flow to the brain, leading to a certain type of dementia (vascular dementia) (3).

4.3 WE ARE WHAT WE DIDN'T EAT

In the United States nowadays health problems and chronic illnesses either wholly or partly attributable to our Standard American Diet (SAD), i.e., the so-called Western Pattern Diet, represent by far the most serious threat to public health: 65% of adults 20 years old or older are either overweight or obese, and the estimated number of deaths ascribable to obesity is close to 300,000 per year. More than 64 million Americans have one or more types of cardiovascular disease, which represents the leading cause of mortality in the United States (38.5% of all deaths). Fifty million Americans are hypertensive; 11 million have Type 2 diabetes and 37 million adults maintain high-risk total cholesterol concentrations (240 milligrams [mg]/deciliter [dL]) (4).

What exactly is the said-to-be-unhealthy Western Pattern Diet and how does it contribute to hypertension?

The Western Pattern Diet is a modern dietary pattern that is generally characterized by high intakes of pre-packaged foods, refined grains, red meat, processed meat, high-sugar drinks, candy and sweets, fried foods, conventionally-raised animal products, butter and other high-fat dairy products, eggs, potatoes, corn (and high-fructose corn syrup), and it is low in intake of fruits, vegetables, whole grains, pasture-raised animal products, fish, nuts and seeds (5).

The US Department of Agriculture (USDA) Dietary Guidelines for Americans defines the diet as being too low in fresh fruits and vegetables, whole grains, lean protein and healthy oils, and too high in red meat, high-fat dairy products, processed and fast foods, refined carbohydrates, added sugars, salt and calories. Furthermore, the amount of omega-3 polyunsaturated fats in the Western diet has declined while the consumption of omega-6 fatty acids (FAs) has increased substantially. This is due to the development and use of vegetable and seed oils in our food supply.

The USDA advises Americans that vegetable and seed oils (olive oil, soybean oil, canola oil and sunflower oil) are healthy fats, but it neglects to mention that these oils are highly processed industrial products. Not only are they high in potentially inflammatory omega-6 FAs, but their production process introduces other toxins such as hexane and pesticides into the final product (6). Almost all processed foods contain one or more vegetable oils.

But in the end, it is the *overabundance* of omega-6-rich oils in comparison to the under-abundance of omega-3 FAs in the standard American (Western) diet that tilts it toward being pro-hypertension and pro-inflammatory. That, coupled with the likelihood of widespread omega-3 deficiency and its consequences. Such a deficiency has been reported by a number of sources. Omega-3 polyunsaturated FA deficiency during pregnancy can cause hypertension in the later life of the offspring.

The antioxidant diet of a mother (a rat, in this case) affects blood pressure later in the life of the offspring. A study examined the effect of different sources of alpha-linolenic acid, such as canola oil or flaxseed oil, in the prevention of hypertension induced by an omega-3 FA-deficient diet. It was published in 2010, in the journal *Hypertension Research*. The investigators reported an experimental animal model study (rats) that showed that even a low omega-3 FA diet in the "mothers" can affect later blood pressure in the offspring (7).

Research links an imbalance in the omega-6 to omega-3 FAs ratio to a long list of chronic diseases, including heart disease and Type 2 diabetes (8). But omega-6s, *per se*, are cardioprotective (9). Yet it is because the Western diet is also poor in antioxidants overall that it also contributes to its promotion of hypertension and cardiovascular disorders.

Contrary to what was said about antioxidants in connection with ORAC (you may recall from the last chapter), the National Center for Complementary and Integrative Health of the National Institutes of Health (NIH) now tells us that consuming greater amounts of antioxidant-rich foods might actually help to protect against diseases (10). A diet naturally rich in antioxidants might help prevent the development of hypertension.

In fact, a study published in 2007 in the *Journal of the American College of Nutrition* aimed to determine whether consumption of a meal of different fruits or berries increases plasma antioxidant capacity measured as ORAC in blood.

Plasma ORAC measures were obtained after participants consumed a *single meal* of berries/fruits, i.e., blueberry, dried plum, dried plum juice, grape, cherry, kiwifruit and strawberry. It was found that after consuming certain berries and fruits such as blueberries, mixed grape and kiwifruit, that plasma ORAC rose while by comparison consuming foods containing no antioxidants resulted in a decline in plasma ORAC (11). What's more, in a study published in the *Nutrition Journal* in 2019, the risk of hypertension was found to be inversely associated with the antioxidant capacity of the diet, in a large prospective cohort of women. This suggested that promoting a diet naturally rich in antioxidants might help prevent the development of hypertension (12).

There are many more clinical studies that underscore the role of antioxidants in diet to maintain normal blood pressure, and that antioxidant-poor diets promote hypertension.

But does the same outcome apply to the intake of omega-3 FAs? For the most part, and for obvious ethical reasons, the experimental studies that show that you can induce hypertension with an omega-3-deficient diet have been conducted on animal models (rats usually). But there are clinical studies.

Omega-3 FAs reduce blood pressure even better in people with elevated blood pressure than in those with high-normal blood pressure. A study titled "Whole blood omega-3 fatty acid concentrations are inversely associated with blood pressure in young, healthy adults," was published in the *Journal of Hypertension* in 2018. The Omega-3 Index was determined in whole blood in participants known not to have cardiovascular disease, diabetes or a BMI greater than 35 kilograms (kg)/square meter (m^2). It was found that the median Omega-3 Index was 4.58%. Compared with individuals in the lowest Omega-3 Index quartile, individuals in the highest quartile had a significantly lower systolic and diastolic blood pressure.

The investigators concluded that a higher Omega-3 Index is significantly associated with clinically relevant lower systolic and diastolic blood pressure in individuals with normal blood pressure, and they propose that diets rich in omega-3 FAs may be an appropriate primary prevention of hypertension strategy (13). But what if one is already hypertensive? It turns out that omega-3s are even more effective in lowering blood pressure in persons with hypertension. This was shown in a study published in the journal *Cellular and Molecular Biology* in 2010. The investigators found that omega-3 FAs reduce blood pressure even more in hypertensive patients and those with high-normal blood pressure if they are given at least 3–4 g/day (14).

Increased marine omega-3 FA intake from fish consumption is recommended as a part of non-pharmacological treatment of hypertension. A review published in the *British Journal of Nutrition* in 2012 found that high doses of omega-3 FAs (greater than 3 g/day) produce a small but significant decrease in blood pressure, especially systolic blood pressure, in older and hypertensive people (15). In the following study, marine omega-3s are an alternative to antihypertensive medications in newly diagnosed patients.

That clinical study, published in 2017 in the journal *Nutrition Research*, aimed to determine whether higher habitual fish intake and omega-3 FA plasma levels were associated with lower blood pressure, and being less likely to receive antihypertensive medication after a one-year follow-up. It was found that in patients with newly diagnosed, untreated hypertension, regular fish consumption was accompanied by lower blood pressure suggesting that an increase in marine omega-3 FA intake should be a part of non-pharmacological treatment of hypertension (16).

4.4 BLOOD PRESSURE AND THE OMEGA-3 INDEX (O3I)

The Omega-3 Index (O3I), as noted previously, is often used to evaluate the body levels of omega-3 FAs. It does that by assessing the levels of all FAs in red blood cell membranes. Then, it determines the proportion of omega-3s, given as a percentage.

In the following chapters, it will be suggested that one test for level of omega-3s before starting a high omega-3 diet plan and then again after some time has passed, to see how successful the diet plan was in raising the omega-3 level. So, how long should one wait to retest?

Dr W.S. Harris, a pioneer in the development of the O3I (https:// omegaquant.com /about/), suggests that

> people wait to retest for 4 months, the time it takes for red blood cells, on which the test is based, to all be replaced. One may, however, certainly see a rise in the Omega 3 Index (O3I) by 1 month, more at 2, etc. until at 4 months one is pretty close to being in a new steady state. [By his calculations,] if a person starts at 4% O3I, it will take 1200-1500 mg of additional EPA+DHA to get to 8% on average. Some people need more; others less, but that's a good starting point. (With permission.)

Foods enriched with algae-sourced omega-3 FAs may serve as alternative dietary sources of omega-3 FAs. In a study published in 2020 in the journal *Scientific Reports*, the authors tell us that the very prevalent diets low in seafood omega-3 polyunsaturated FAs have recently been ranked as the sixth most important dietary risk factor, incurring 1.5 million deaths, and 33 million disability-adjusted life-years worldwide. What's more, wild oily fish stocks are not in sufficient supply to feed the world's population, and levels of eicosapentaenoic acid (EPA) and docosahexaenoic acid (DHA) in farmed fish have more than halved in the last 20 years.

Therefore, they conducted a study wherein healthy normotensive adults were given at least three portions per week of omega-3 FA-enriched (or control) chicken meat, and to eat at least three omega-3 FA-enriched (or control) eggs/week, for 6 months. They found that regular consumption of omega-3 FA-enriched chicken meat and eggs significantly increased the red cell O3I compared to a group that ate both control foods. The number of participants with a very high-risk O3I was more than halved in those participants who ate enriched foods. And, most important, eating the enriched foods resulted in significant and clinically relevant reductions in diastolic blood pressure.

The investigators concluded that foods naturally enriched with algae-sourced omega-3 FAs may serve as alternative dietary sources of these essential nutrients. Unlike many lifestyle interventions, long-term population health benefits should not depend on the willingness of individuals to make long-lasting dietary changes that are difficult, but instead should depend on the ready availability of a range of commonly eaten and relatively inexpensive, omega-3 FA-enriched foods (17).

Parenthetically, according to the Flax Council of Canada, Omega-3-fortified eggs are fortified by feeding flax to laying hens. These eggs contain the essential omega-3 FA, alpha-linolenic (ALA), plus two other omega-3 FAs: EPA and DHA (18). Omega-3-enriched eggs provide a much higher amount of omega-3 than regular eggs, but the total can vary widely between brands. For instance:

Brand	Omega-3 Content per Large Egg
Christopher	660 mg
4 Grain	150 mg
Sauder's Eggs	325 mg
Eggland's	115 mg

4.5 OMEGA-3 FATTY ACIDS REDUCE THE INFLAMMATION PROCESS IN ATHEROSCLEROSIS

So, in the spirit of John Locke, let's clear the ground a little and "remove some of the rubbish which lies in the way to knowledge." It is a common message that atherosclerosis "clogs arteries" and that it can cut off blood circulation in parts of the body or in the brain. The common image is sludge coating the inner surface of a blood vessel. Well, it is true that atherosclerosis can clog arteries, but it does it differently than the way it is commonly understood to do. It is important to clear this up because that underscores the value of omega-3s (see Figure 4.1).

This figure comes from a clinical study titled "Mechanisms, functional consequences, and potential therapeutics for cellular senescence." What this title actually says is that our body ages when our cells develop atherosclerosis, this is why that happens, and here is what we can do about it. This appeared in 2012 in the journal *Circulation Research*—the official journal of the American Heart Association.

The space on the top of the figure, where it says "blood flow," is the inside of the blood vessel, i.e., the *lumen*. The wall of the blood vessel encroaches into the lumen, narrowing it as the vessel swells with the formation of atherosclerosis. This is what

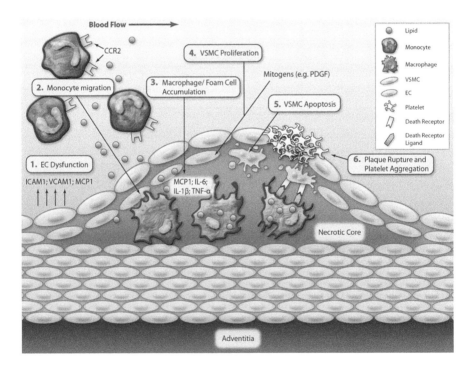

FIGURE 4.1 Schematic of the formation of atherosclerosis and an unstable atherosclerotic plaque. (Illustration: Cosmocyte/Ben Smith. Source: Wang and Bennett. 2012. *Circulation Research* (19). With permission.)

they are talking about when they say that atherosclerosis narrows the blood vessels—it's about that inward bulge. It is not about anything plastering the inside of the vessel as is commonly thought.

Plaque formation begins with monocytes, a type of white blood cell, maturing into macrophage foam cells as they gorge on oxidized lipids.

For some reason, the authors do not label the green cells, i.e., the endothelium. Notice that as plaque forms, it distances the endothelium from the rest of the blood vessel. It actually separates it from the other portions of the blood vessel wall.

Now here's the problem: The endothelium cannot derive oxygen or nutrients from the bloodstream. You may recall that blood vessels have their own blood vessels, the *vasa vasorum*, on which they depend for oxygen and nutrients. But if you distance the endothelium from the remainder of the vessel walls you also distance it from the vasa vasorum that run through it, bringing its only source of oxygen and nutrients. So even before atherosclerosis is so advanced that it can result in rupture and blood clot formation (thrombosis), it has already for some time seriously damaged the endothelium by distancing it from its oxygen supply, thus reducing that supply.

So, the SAD, aka the Western Pattern Diet, offers a two-pronged approach to damaging the endothelium: First, a high-salt, high-sugar diet damages the glycocalyx exposing the endothelium to blood borne ROS hazards. This damages the endothelium from the outside. Then, a high-saturated fat, low-omega-3 FA, low-antioxidant diet enhances plaque formation within the vessel wall, starving the endothelium. Double whammy!

So, let's see how plaque formation can be prevented by omega-3 FAs, or even reversed if it has already begun to form.

4.6 OMEGA-3s MAY PREVENT ATHEROSCLEROSIS AND STABILIZE, EVEN REDUCE, PLAQUE

A review of relevant research titled "The effects of fish oil on cardiovascular diseases: systematical evaluation and recent advance" published in the journal *Frontiers in Cardiovascular Medicine*, in 2022, concluded that omega-3 FAs are anti-inflammatory, antioxidant, improve endothelial function, reduce the risk of blood clots and lower levels of blood lipids (20).

The O3I correlates with atherosclerosis status. The aim of a study published in the journal *Atherosclerosis*, in 2019, was to determine a target level of EPA and DHA that would prevent progression of coronary artery plaque. Participants with stable coronary artery disease receiving statins were given high-dose EPA and DHA (3.36 grams (g) daily) for 30 months, or a control group that received no supplemental omega-3 for the same time period. Participants on the EPA and DHA supplement had significantly increased plasma EPA and DHA levels. Total plaque progression was prevented in participants with plasma O3I ≥ 4%, whereas those in the lowest quartile (<3.43%) had significant progression of fibrous, calcified and total plaque (21).

4.7 OMEGA-3 FATTY ACIDS CAN REDUCE CORONARY ARTERY PLAQUE

It is reported in a study published in the *Journal of the Federation of American Societies of Experimental Biology* (FASEB), in 2021, that a group of patients with stable coronary artery disease treated with statins were given 3.36 g daily of EPA and DHA, whereas a control group received no supplemental EPA/DHA. Coronary plaque volume was measured at the start and at a 30-month follow-up. It was found that patients with low plasma EPA + DHA levels at the end of the study period had significant plaque progression, whereas those with high plasma EPA + DHA levels at the end of the study period had significant plaque regression. Their findings suggest that inflammation plays a significant role in coronary artery disease and that EPA and DHA benefit coronary artery disease patients by their anti-inflammatory effects (22).

There have been numerous studies of the benefits of flaxseed in atherosclerosis, but most are conducted on animal models—rabbits mostly. These studies should not be discounted just because they are rabbit models, since the rabbit develops and suffers from atherosclerosis as we do. To wit …

4.8 LIGNANS IN FLAXSEED SLOW PROGRESSION OF ATHEROSCLEROSIS

An experimental animal model study published in the *Journal of Cardiovascular Pharmacology and Therapeutics,* in 2019, aimed to determine whether flax lignan complex could slow the progression of already developed atherosclerosis in four groups of rabbits: group I, regular diet (2 months); group II, 0.25% cholesterol diet (2 months); group III, 0.25% cholesterol diet (4 months); group IV, 0.25% cholesterol diet (2 months) followed by 0.25% cholesterol diet plus flax lignan complex (2 months). Atherosclerosis in group II was associated with elevated lipids and increased oxidative stress. Significant areas of the aortic surfaces from group II, group III and group IV held atherosclerotic plaques. Group IV rabbits had 40% more atherosclerotic lesions than group II but 31% fewer lesions than group III. The flax lignan complex-induced reduction in the progression of atherosclerosis and was associated with reductions in oxidative stress.

The investigators concluded that flax lignan complex was effective in slowing down the progression of atherosclerosis by 31%, and this effect was associated with a reduction in oxidative stress[*] (23).

So, omega-3s from fish plus lignans from flaxseed can prevent, retard and even reverse atherosclerosis. This benefits the endothelium, thus preserving NO availability essential in blood vessel and heart function.

---

[*] Oxidative stress was measured in this study by levels of *malondialdehyde* (MDA), a by-product of ROS, described in a previous chapter in connection with "measuring" free radicals.

4.9 TYPE 2 DIABETES—ANTS KNOW IT LONG BEFORE YOU DO

Want to know how to detect diabetes? Here's a simple test developed hundreds of years ago. Around 500 BC, Hindu healers poured the urine of people suspected of having diabetes on the ground to see if ants were attracted to it. If they were, they were said to have a condition called "madhumeha," or "honey urine." Ants "know" when there's sugar in urine. It is recommended that you don't try this at home.

People with diabetes have unhealthy elevated levels of sugar, i.e., glucose, in their blood and it shows up in their urine. The reason is that their body either doesn't produce enough insulin, or it is insulin resistant. Lingering elevated blood glucose combines with oxygen (oxidizes) free radicals in blood to form ROS that cause inflammation and, according to a 2018 report in the journal *Arteriosclerosis, Thrombosis and Vascular Biology*, first damage the glycocalyx by shedding some of its components and then damages the endothelium (24). This is why elevated glucose creates havoc in virtually all organs in the body.

Since all organs in the body rely on blood circulation for oxygen, nutrients, carbon dioxide and waste removal, attacking the endothelium and jeopardizing NO formation is a really bad idea. We will briefly and *pro forma* list the early signs of Type 2 diabetes and then described the damage that it can do to organs in the body, and how omega-3s can come to the rescue.

Type 2 is the most common type of diabetes. There are about 29 million people in the United States with Type 2 diabetes, and another 84 million have pre-diabetes, meaning their blood glucose is high, but not high enough to be said to be diabetes. Signs and symptoms of Type 2 diabetes often develop slowly. In fact, one can have Type 2 diabetes for years and not know it. According to the Mayo Clinic website, when signs and symptoms are present, they may include:

- Increased thirst.
- Frequent urination.
- Increased hunger.
- Unintended weight loss.
- Fatigue.
- Blurred vision.
- Slow-healing sores.
- Frequent infections.
- Numbness or tingling in the hands or feet.
- Areas of darkened skin, usually in the armpits and neck (25).

Type 2 diabetes causes numerous cardiovascular disorders (26), as well as other debilitating conditions including:

- Heart and blood vessel disease (see Chapter 3).
- Nerve damage (neuropathy).
- Kidney disease (see Chapter 5).
- Eye damage.

- Slow healing.
- Hearing impairment.
- Skin conditions.

Some of these will be described below. But first, do omega-3 FAs benefit people with Type 2 diabetes *per se*? The clinical and research findings are equivocal. For instance, a 2018 report in the journal *Cardiovascular Diabetology* concludes that omega-3 FA supplementation lowers blood lipids, reduces inflammation and improves blood glucose levels (27). And, investigators reported in the journal *PLoS One*, in 2015, that the ratio of EPA/DHA and early intervention with omega-3 FAs may have beneficial effects on glucose control and lipid levels, "which may serve as a dietary reference for clinicians or nutritionists who manage diabetic patients" (28).

4.10 LONG-TERM INTAKE OF OMEGA-3 FATTY ACIDS FROM FISH LOWERS THE RISK OF DEVELOPING TYPE 2 DIABETES

A study published in the journal *Diabetes Care* in 2014 aimed to determine whether serum omega-3 FAs EPA, DPA, DHA and ALA, affected the risk of Type 2 diabetes in middle-aged and older Finnish men.

A total of 2,212 men from the prospective, population-based Kuopio Ischemic Heart Disease Risk Factor study, aged 42–60 years and free of Type 2 diabetes at baseline in 1984–1989, were followed and re-examined at 4, 11 and 20 years. During an average follow-up of 19.3 years, 422 of the men (19%) developed Type 2 diabetes. Those in the highest versus the lowest serum EPA + DPA + DHA quartile had a 33% significant lower risk for developing Type 2 diabetes. The investigators concluded omega-3 FA concentration, an objective biomarker for fish intake, was associated with long-term lower risk of Type 2 diabetes (29).

Not everyone is onboard. A 2008 report in the *Cochrane Database of Systematic Reviews* concluded that omega-3 FA supplementation in Type 2 diabetes lowers triglycerides and very low density lipoprotein (VLDL) cholesterol, but it has no significant effect on blood glucose control (30).

There are two main issues that people with Type 2 diabetes face. First, the early signs of elevated blood sugar (glucose) are not clear cut. It is only when they become more severe or more frequent that one may take notice of them, and even then it is not clear what the problem is because there is no general awareness that the cluster of symptoms portends diabetes. Therefore, most people learn about their condition first when it is diagnosed in a routine medical exam.

Second, because the signs may be somewhat troubling, but they seem to cause no discernible problems—at first—there is a tendency to underestimate the severity of chronically elevated blood glucose. For the same reason, noncompliance with medications—which work reasonably well to control blood glucose levels—is a feature in the epidemiology of this disease: According to a report in the journal *Patient Preference and Adherence* in 2016, at least 45% of patients with Type 2 diabetes fail to achieve adequate blood glucose control, i.e., an hemoglobin A1c (HbA1c) less than 7%. The HbA1c test measures the amount of blood sugar (glucose) attached to your hemoglobin.

One of the major contributing factors is poor medication adherence. That is a major reason for the diabetes-related disorders described below (31).

4.11 OMEGA-3 FATTY ACIDS AND HEART AND BLOOD VESSEL DISEASE IN TYPE 2 DIABETES

According to *Web*MD, heart disease is common in people with diabetes. The National Heart Association reported in 2012 that 65% of people with diabetes will die from some sort of heart disease or stroke. In general, in people with diabetes, the risks of death from heart disease and stroke are more than twice as high as in normal people. While all people with diabetes have an increased chance of developing heart disease, the condition is more common in those with Type 2 diabetes. In fact, heart disease is the number one cause of death among people with Type 2 diabetes (32).

Do you remember the phrase "It's the economy, stupid" coined by James Carville in 1992 in connection with the Bill Clinton campaign? Well, having read this book so far, you may be saying to yourself as you read about the damage done by diabetes to the blood vessels, the heart and the eyes, "It's the endothelium, stupid." Omega-3 FAs sustain heart and blood vessel function by their beneficial effects on endothelium. That was made clear in a previous chapter.

4.12 OMEGA-3 FATTY ACIDS AND PERIPHERAL NEUROPATHY

According to the Mayo Clinic website, diabetic neuropathy is a type of nerve damage that affects as many as 50% of people with diabetes. It is seen most often in the legs and feet. Depending on the affected nerves, diabetic neuropathy symptoms can range from pain and numbness in the legs and feet to problems with the digestive system, urinary tract, blood vessels and heart. Some people have mild symptoms, but in others it can be quite painful and disabling (33). Can omega-3s play a beneficial role in diabetic neuropathy?

Fish oil supplements can restore the condition of nerves damaged by diabetes (in mice). In May 2015, *Science Daily* reported that "Fish oil may help with diabetic neuropathy." The article tells us that "A new study in the *Journal of Neurophysiology*, however, introduces a new alternative, omega-3 fatty acids found in fish oil. The study shows that fish oil supplements can restore the condition of nerves damaged from diabetes in mice." But similar results have been reported in connection with the benefits of omega-3 FAs in people with diabetic neuropathy. For instance, a report in 2018 in the journal *Current Diabetes Reviews* concludes that dietary enrichment with omega-3 FAs contained in fish oil may be a beneficial treatment for diabetic neuropathy (34).

Omega-3 FA treatment can lower the chances that kidney disease, common in Type 2 diabetes patients, will progress to kidney failure. Many other studies have shown that omega-3 FAs could reduce the severity of neuropathy in patients with Type 2 diabetes mellitus. The following study shows that it also benefits kidney function. For instance, in 1996, the *Journal of Diabetes Complications* reported a study aimed to investigate the efficacy of a new, highly purified product from natural omega-3 FA EPA, after oral administration at a dose of 1,800 mg/day for 48 weeks in patients with Type 2 diabetes mellitus.

It was found that the treatment improved the clinical symptom of coldness and numbness. There was also a significant decrease of serum triglycerides as well a significant decreased excretion of albumin in urine. Treatment that lowers the urine albumin level may lower the chances that kidney disease, common in Type 2 diabetes patients, will progress to kidney failure. It was concluded that the present form of omega-3, i.e., EPA-E, has significant beneficial effects on diabetic neuropathy and serum lipids as well as other diabetic complications such as kidney disease, nephropathy and blood vessel disease (35).

4.13 OMEGA-3 FATTY ACIDS BENEFITS IN TYPE 2 DIABETES EYE DAMAGE (RETINOPATHY)—THE SECRET REVEALED

One of the major debilitating complications of Type 2 diabetes is potentially blinding damage to the eyes caused by the chronic elevated blood sugar. Blood vessels in the retina, the area in the back of the eye where vision is discerned, leak causing detachment of parts of, or all of the retina from the eyeball wall to which it is attached.

Based on a review of websites that address this issue for the public, the Mayo Clinic website included that one would have to arrive at the conclusion that the actual basis of this eye disease, namely endothelium damage by ROS stems from chronic elevated blood glucose, is a carefully guarded secret. Doctors don't tend to tell you that. But now you know. And, the retina, by the way, is rich in omega-3 FAs which are important anti-inflammatory antioxidants that Nature put there for a reason.

The endothelium damage basis of diabetic retinopathy is underscored in a report published in the journal *Frontiers in Endocrinology* in 2020. We learn in this report that diabetic retinopathy, which affects retinal function, resulting in severe loss of vision, is caused by a number of factors and here is a sample from those they cite:

- *Advanced glycosylation end products*: A key factor in diabetes is an increase in a process in which glucose and other sugars attach to proteins, causing proteins throughout the body to become dysfunctional.
- *Pro-inflammatory cytokines*: These substances are secreted by the immune system and promote inflammation.
- *Oxidative stress* is the cost of the balance between ROS and antioxidant defenses (36).

This boils down to impaired endothelial function and NO unavailability.

In middle-aged and older Type 2 diabetes sufferers, at least 500 mg/day of dietary omega-3 FAs (easily achievable with two weekly servings of oily fish) lowers the risk of diabetic retinopathy. The study that reported these findings was published in the *Journal of the American Medical Association—Ophthalmology*, in 2016. It aimed to determine whether omega-3 FA intake decreases the incidence of sight-threatening diabetic retinopathy in persons with Type 2 diabetes who are older than 55 years. The participants, followed up for about 6 years, who followed the ≥500 mg/day omega-3 FAs recommendation, showed a 48% reduced risk of incident sight-threatening diabetic retinopathy, an outcome significantly better than that of the control group that did not meet that FA intake.

The investigators concluded that in middle-aged and older individuals with Type 2 diabetes, intake of at least 500 mg/day of dietary omega-3 FAs, easily achievable with two weekly servings of oily fish, is associated with a decreased risk of sight-threatening diabetic retinopathy (37).

4.14 OMEGA-3 FATTY ACIDS IMPROVE DIABETIC SLOW WOUND-HEALING

One of the most common complications of diabetes is chronic wounds, primarily in the feet. Diabetes inhibits the body's natural wound-healing capabilities which means chronic wounds can quickly become severe and develop infections if left untreated. What can omega-3 FAs contribute to healing?

Omega-3 supplementation helps in wound healing, according to a report in 2017 in the *Journal of Diabetes Complications*. Omega-3 FA supplementation was given to patients with diabetic foot ulcer for 12 weeks. There followed a significant reduction in ulcer length, width and depth. Omega-3 supplementation also had a beneficial effect on insulin metabolism. It significantly reduced serum insulin concentration and serum high sensitivity C-Reactive Protein, a marker of inflammation. There was also a significant increase in plasma total antioxidant capacity and glutathione concentrations (38).

REFERENCES

1. Ciszek B, Cieślicki K, Krajewski P, and SK Piechnik. 2013. Critical pressure for arterial Wall rupture in major human cerebral arteries. *Stroke*, Nov; 44 (11), 3226–3228. DOI: 10.1161/STROKEAHA.113.002370.
2. Kalinowski L, Dobrucki IT, and T Malinski. 2004. Race-specific differences in endothelial function: predisposition of African Americans to vascular diseases. *Circulation*, Jun 1; 109(21): 2511–2517. DOI: 10.1161/01.CIR.0000129087. 81352.7A.
3. https://www.mayoclinic.org/diseases-conditions/high-blood-pressure/symptoms-causes/syc-20373410; accessed 1/28/22.
4. Cordain L, Eaton SB, Sebastian A, Mann N, Lindeberg S, Watkins BA, O'Keefe JH, and J Brand-Miller. 2005. Origins and evolution of the Western diet: health implications for the 21st century. *American Journal of Clinical Nutrition*, 81: 341–354. DOI: 10.1093/ajcn.81.2.341.
5. Halton TL, Willett WC, Liu S, Manson JE, Stampfer MJ, Hu FB. 2006. Potato and french fry consumption and risk of type 2 diabetes in women. *American Journal of Clinical Nutrition*, 83(2): 284–290. DOI: 10.1093/ajcn/83.2.284.
6. https://extension.psu.edu/processing-edible-oils; accessed 1/29/22.
7. Begg DP, Sinclair AJ, Stahl LA, Premaratna SD, Hafandi A, Jois M, and RS Weisinger. 2010. Hypertension induced by omega-3 polyunsaturated fatty acid deficiency is alleviated by alpha-linolenic acid regardless of dietary source. *Hypertension Research*, Aug; 33(8): 808–813. DOI: 10.1038/hr.2010.84.

8. Simopoulos AP. 2008. The importance of the omega-6/omega-3 fatty acid ratio in cardiovascular disease and other chronic diseases. *Experimental Biology and Medicine (Maywood)*, Jun; 233(6): 674–688. DOI: 10.3181/0711-MR-311.
9. Yeung J, Tourdot BE, Adili R, Green AR, Freedman CJ, Fernandez-Perez P, Yu J, Holman TR, and M Holinstat. 2016. 12(S)-HETrE, a 12-lipoxygenase oxylipin of dihomo-γ-linolenic acid, inhibits thrombosis via gas signaling in platelets. *Arteriosclerosis, Thrombosis, and Vascular Biology*, Oct; 36(10):2068–2077. DOI: 10.1161/ATVBAHA.116.308050.
10. https://www. nccih.nih. gov/health/antioxidants-in-depth; accessed 1/29/22.
11. Prior RL, Gu L, Wu X, Jacob RA, Sotoudeh G, Kader AA, and RA Cook. 2007. Plasma antioxidant capacity changes following a meal as a measure of the ability of a food to alter in vivo antioxidant status. *Journal of the American College of Nutrition*, 26(2): 170–181. https://doi.org/10.1080/07315724.2007.10719599.
12. Villaverde P, Lajous M, MacDonald, CJ, Fagherazzi G, Bonnet F, and M-C Boutron-Ruault . 2019. High dietary total antioxidant capacity is associated with a reduced risk of hypertension in French women. *Nutrition Journal*, 18(31). https://doi.org/ 10.1186/s12937-019-0456-0.
13. Filipovic MG, Aeschbacher S, Reiner MF, Simona Stivala S, Gobbato S, Bonetti N, Risch M, Risch L, Camici GC, Luescher TF, von Schacky C, Conen D, and JH Beera. 2018. Whole blood omega-3 fatty acid concentrations are inversely associated with blood pressure in young, healthy adults. *Journal of Hypertension*, Jul; 36(7): 1548–1554. DOI: 10.1097/HJH.0000000000001728.
14. Mori TA. 2010. Omega-3 fatty acids and blood pressure. *Cellular and Molecular Biology (Noisy-le-grand)*, Feb 25; 56(1): 83–92. PMID: 20196972
15. Cabo J, Alonso R, and P Mata. 2012. Omega-3 fatty acids and blood pressure. *British Journal of Nutrition*, Jun; 107(Suppl 2): S195–S200. DOI: 10.1017/S0007114512001584.
16. Bagge CN, Strandhave C, Skov CM, Svensson M, Schmidt EB, and JH Christensen. 2017. Marine n-3 polyunsaturated fatty acids affect the blood pressure control in patients with newly diagnosed hypertension - a 1-year follow-up study. *Nutrition Research*, Feb; 38: 71–78. DOI: 10.1016/j.nutres.2017.02.009.
17. Stanton AV, James K, Brennan MM, O'Donovan F, Buskandar F, Shortall K, El-Sayed T, Jean Kennedy J, Hayes H, Fahey AG, Pender N, Thom SAM, Moran N, Williams DJ, and E Dolan. 2020. Omega-3 index and blood pressure responses to eating foods naturally enriched with omega-3 polyunsaturated fatty acids: a randomized controlled trial. *Scientific Reports*, 2020; 10: 15444. DOI: 10.1038/s41598-020-71801-5.
18. https://flaxcouncil.ca/resources/nutrition/general-nutrition-information/flax-in-a-vegetarian-diet/omega-3-enriched-eggs/#:~:text=Omega%2D3%20eggs%20are%20eggs,)%20and%20docosahexaenoic%20(DHA); accessed 4.2.22.
19. Wang JC, and M Bennett. 2012. Aging and atherosclerosis. Mechanisms, functional consequences, and potential therapeutics for cellular senescence. *Circulation Research*, Jul 6; 111(2): 111:245–259. DOI: 10.1161/CIRCRESAHA. 111.261388.
20. Liao J, Xiong Q, Yin Y, Ling Z, and S Chen. 2022. The effects of fish oil on cardiovascular diseases: Systematical evaluation and recent advance. *Frontiers in Cardiovascular Medicine*, Jan 5; 8: 802306. DOI: 10.3389/fcvm.2021.802306.
21. Alfaddagh A, Elajami TK, Saleh M, Mohebali D, Bistrian BR, and FK Welty FK. 2019. An omega-3 fatty acid plasma index ≥4% prevents progression of coronary artery plaque in patients with coronary artery disease on statin treatment. *Atherosclerosis*, Jun; 285: 153–162. DOI: 10.1016/j.atherosclerosis.2019.04.213.

22. Welty FK, Schulte F, Alfaddagh A, Elajami TK, Bistrian BR, and M Hardt. 2021. Regression of human coronary artery plaque is associated with a high ratio of (18-hydroxy-eicosapentaenoic acid + resolvin E1) to leukotriene B 4. *FASEB J*, Apr; 35(4): e21448. DOI: 10.1096/fj.202002471R.
23. Prasad K. 2009. Flax lignan complex slows down the progression of atherosclerosis in hyperlipidemic rabbits. *Journal of Cardiovascular Pharmacology and Therapeutics*, March: 38–48. DOI: 10.1177/1074248408330541.
24. Dogné S, Flamion B, and N Caron. 2018. Endothelial glycocalyx as a shield against diabetic vascular complications. Involvement of hyaluronan and hyaluronidases. *Arteriosclerosis, Thrombosis and Vascular Biology*, Jul; 38(7): 1427–1439. DOI: 10.1161/ATVBAHA.118.310839.
25. Mayo Clinic: https://www.mayoclinic.org/diseases-conditions/type-2-diabetes/ symptoms-causes/syc-20351193.
26. Fried R, and RM Carlton. 2018. *Type 2 Diabetes: Cardiovascular and Related Complications and Evidence-Based Complementary Treatments.* CRC Press.
27. O'Mahoney LL, Matu J, Price OJ, Birch KM, Ajjan RA, Farrar D, Tapp R, West DJ, Deighton K, and MD Campbell. 2018. Omega-3 polyunsaturated fatty acids favourably modulate cardiometabolic biomarkers in type 2 diabetes: a meta-analysis and meta-regression of randomized controlled trials. *Cardiovascular Diabetology*, Jul 7; 17(1): 98. DOI: 10.1186/s12933-018-0740-x.
28. Chen C, Yu X, and S Shao. 2015. Effects of omega-3 fatty acid supplementation on glucose control and lipid levels in Type 2 diabetes: A meta-analysis. *PLoS One*, Oct 2; 10(10): e0139565. DOI: 10.1371/journal.pone.0139565.
29. Virtanen JK, Mursu J, Voutilainen S, Uusitupa M, and T-P Tuomainen. 2014. Serum omega-3 polyunsaturated fatty acids and risk of incident type 2 diabetes in men: the Kuopio Ischemic Heart Disease Risk Factor study. *Diabetes Care*, 37(1): 189–196. DOI: 10.2337/dc13-1504.
30. Hartweg J, Perera R, Montori V, Dinneen S, Neil HAW, and A Farmer. 2008. Omega-3 polyunsaturated fatty acids (PUFA) for Type 2 diabetes mellitus. *Cochrane Database of Systematic Reviews*, Jan 23; (1): CD003205. DOI: 10.1002/14651858.CD00 3205.pub2.
31. Polonsky WH, and RR Henry. 2016. Poor medication adherence in type 2 diabetes: recognizing the scope of the problem and its key contributors. *Patient Preference and Adherence*, 10: 1299–1307. DOI: 10.2147/PPA.S106821.
32. https://www.webmd.com/diabetes/heart-blood-disease; accessed 2/5/22.
33. https://www.mayoclinic.org/diseases-conditions/diabetic-neuropathy/symptoms-causes/syc-2037158; accessed 2/5/22.
34. Yorek MA. 2018. Is fish oil a potential treatment for diabetic peripheral neuropathy? *Current Diabetes Reviews*, 14(4): 339–349. DOI: 10.2174/1573399813666 170522155327.
35. Okud Y, Mizutani M, Ogawa M, Sone H, Asano M, Asakura Y, Isaka M, Suzuki S, Kawakami Y, Field JB, and K Yamashita. 1996. Long-term effects of eicosapentaenoic acid on diabetic peripheral neuropathy and serum lipids in patients with type II diabetes mellitus. *Journal of Diabetes Complications*, Sep–Oct; 10(5): 280–287. DOI: 10.1016/1056-8727(95)00081-x.
36. Gui F, You Z, Fu S, Wu H, and Y Zhang. 2020. Endothelial dysfunction in diabetic retinopathy. *Frontiers in Endocrinology (Lausanne)*, 11: 591. DOI: 10.3389/fendo.2020.00591.
37. Sala-Vila A, Díaz-López A, Valls-Pedret C, Cofán M, García-Layana A, Lamuela-Raventós R-M, Castañer O, Zanon-Moreno V, Martinez-Gonzalez MA, Toledo E, Basora J, Salas-Salvadó J, Corella D, Gómez-Gracia E, Fiol M, Estruch R, Lapetra

J, Fitó M, Arós F, Serra-Majem L, Pintó X, Ros E, and the Prevención con Dieta Mediterránea (PREDIMED) Investigators. 2016. Dietary marine ω-3 fatty acids and incident sight-threatening retinopathy in middle-aged and older Individuals with Type 2 diabetes: Prospective investigation from the PREDIMED trial. *JAMA Ophthalmology*, Oct 1; 134(10): 1142–1149. DOI: 10.1001/jamaophthalmol.2016.2906.
38. Khan S. 2017. Diabetic foot ulcer: Omega-3 supplementation helps in wound healing. *Journal of Diabetes Complications*. Aug 22: Univadis. https://www.univadis.co.uk/viewarticle/diabetic-foot-ulcer-omega-3-supplementation-helps-in-wound-healing-546914; accessed 2/6/22.

5 Peripheral Artery Disease, Arthritis, Chronic Kidney Disease, Irritable Bowel Syndrome, Glaucoma, Age-Related Macular Degeneration and Mild Cognitive Impairment in Aging

> Let nothing which can be treated by diet be treated by other means.
>
> —Maimonides

5.1 WHERE'S THE FIRE?

Having read through four chapters so far, if anyone was to ask how it is that omega-6 and omega-3 fatty acids (FAs) in general, and the omega-3s in particular, benefit so many seemingly different medical disorders such as hypertension, atherosclerosis, coronary artery disease, Type 2 diabetes and related disorders, chronic kidney disease, peripheral artery disease, arthritis, glaucoma, age-related macular degeneration and cognitive dysfunction of the elderly, one might be tempted to say, "It's the endothelium! These fatty acids protect the endothelium."

There is little doubt that while these cardiovascular and other disorders seem to be entirely different entities, they are now known to be the consequence of oxidative stress, i.e., the battle between those ROS-things generated by oxygen free radicals made by our own metabolism, slugging it out with the antioxidants (some likewise made by our own bodies, some "imported") to counter them. What is the collateral damage resulting from that struggle? Low-grade chronic systemic inflammation and endothelial dysfunction. Every organ in the body is affected by oxidative stress because it impairs the endothelium of the blood vessels that supplies each of them—from the toes to the eyes. What's more, although this is well known to medical science, nevertheless it is greatly underappreciated in clinical practice.

Here are just a few examples that show just how well this is known:

- Hypertension—"Inflammation can lead to the development of hypertension and that oxidative stress and endothelial dysfunction are involved in the inflammatory cascade" [2014 report in the journal *BioMed Research International* (1)].
- Atherosclerosis—"Inflammation is a process that plays an important role in the initiation and progression of atherosclerosis" [2015 report in the *Central European Journal of Immunology* (2)].
- Coronary Artery Disease—"Although CAD was formerly considered a lipid accumulation-mediated disease, it has now been clearly shown to involve an ongoing inflammatory response" [2014 report in the journal *Cardiology in Review* (3)].
- Type 2 Diabetes—"The emerging role of inflammation in both type 1 and type 2 diabetes (T1D and T2D) pathophysiology and associated metabolic disorders, has generated increasing interest in targeting inflammation to improve prevention and control of the disease" [2019 report in the *European Cardiology Review* (4)].
- Chronic Kidney Disease—"The progression of CKD is closely associated with systemic inflammation and oxidative stress …" [2020 report in the *International Journal of Molecular Sciences* (5)].
- Peripheral artery disease—"Several inflammatory markers play a predictive role in PAD. The best studied is CRP, and the American Heart Association has endorsed its use as an independent marker of increased risk of cardiovascular events" [2010 report in the journal *Circulation* (6)].
- Glaucoma—The website UC San Diego Health, citing a publication in the July 14, 2014, *Proceedings of the National Academy of Sciences*, reported that "Our research is the first to show an inflammatory mechanism by which high ocular pressure causes vision loss in acute glaucoma patients" (7).
- Macular Degeneration—"Elevated levels of markers of systemic inflammation … and higher levels of markers of oxidative stress and endothelial dysfunction …" [2014 report in the *Journal of the American Medical Association (JAMA)—Ophthalmology* (8)].
- Cognitive Impairment in Aging—"Aging is characterized by a progressive increase in neuroinflammation, which contributes to cognitive impairment, associated with aging and age-related neurodegenerative diseases …" [2018 report in the journal *Frontiers in Aging Neuroscience* (9)].

All chronic disorders, no matter how different they appear to be, have one thing in common: chronic low-grade inflammation. And, most importantly, the omega FAs, especially the omega-3s, are anti-inflammatory. So, it shouldn't really matter to the ordinary person whether inflammation causes atherosclerosis, or whether atherosclerosis causes inflammation—likely both—but that, bottom line, you can gain huge improvements in both of them by consuming flax and oily fish.

But if you ask a medical scientist why oxidative stress could result in such different disorder entities, they would probably answer: *genes* expressing themselves. We are all genetically similar but also sufficiently different so that events inside and outside the body are dealt with differently. While we can't control the genetics with which we were born, we CAN control the foodstuffs we ingest and, depending on the conscious choices we make, these can improve (or worsen) the expression of our genes.

5.2 PERIPHERAL ARTERY DISEASE AND CLAUDICATION

Peripheral artery, or vascular, disease (PAD) in the legs or lower extremities results from the narrowing or blockage of the blood vessels in the legs, impeding blood circulation in the limbs. It is primarily caused by atherosclerosis. Risk factors include aging, heart disease, diabetes and smoking—bottom line, according to a 2002 publication in the *European Heart Journal Supplements*, blood vessel endothelial dysfunction (10). Symptoms may include leg pain, particularly when walking, and claudication, which is cramping pain in the legs induced by exercise.

It is important to understand that one develops PAD in the context of atherosclerosis affecting much of the rest of the body as well. In other words, the process of plaque formation does not single out the legs. The American Heart Association (AHA) likens PAD to coronary heart disease and cautions that people with this condition have a higher risk of coronary artery disease, heart attack and stroke as well (11).

Although it has been around for quite some time, there is a test gaining popularity in the assessment of blood flow impairment in the limbs. It is the ankle-brachial index test and it is now recommended by the AHA (12).

5.3 THE ANKLE-BRACHIAL INDEX (ABI)

The ankle-brachial index (ABI) is the ratio of the systolic blood pressure at the ankle to the systolic blood pressure at the brachial artery in the upper arm. It is one of the most widely available markers of atherosclerosis and least expensive to perform. And, by the way, there is also a modified version of it—which we will describe below—that one can do at home and, while it may not be quite as accurate as if it were done in the office of a healthcare provider, if sufficient care is taken, it may be quite adequate to help to determine one's blood circulation status.

The website *Diabetes Self-Management* makes the following recommendations: First, the person lies down for about 10 minutes to equalize the effect of gravity on blood pressure in the arms and legs. Then a blood pressure cuff and/or a Doppler probe (which uses sound waves to detect blood flow) is used to measure blood pressure in the arms and at the ankles (Figure 5.1).

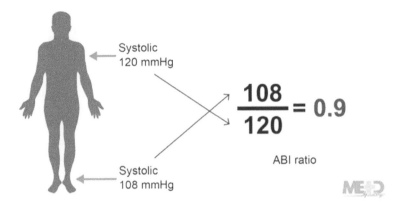

FIGURE 5.1 The Ankle-Brachial Index is the ratio of the blood pressure in the arm to the blood pressure in the leg. (From Medmastery GmbH. With permission.)

(A Doppler is not necessary; an electronic self-inflating cuff will do.) While lying down, face up, the blood pressure cuff is placed over the artery in the arm and inflated. Note the blood pressure. Then it is placed over the artery in the leg and inflated. Note the blood pressure.

Figure 5.2 shows where to place the cuff. The sensor in the cuff goes over the artery. Inflation is allowed to cycle and when it ends, the blood pressure (BP) reading is recorded. This procedure is followed for the right and left arm and leg.

The index is calculated as follows:

ABI = ankle systolic pressure/brachial systolic pressure

The higher of the systolic readings of the left and right arm brachial artery, and the higher of the two ankle systolic values, is used as the basis of the ABI (13, 14). Generally, ABI scores should be interpreted as shown in Table 5.1.

Clinical studies have shown that the sensitivity of the ABI is about 90% with a corresponding 98% specificity for detecting serious abnormal narrowing in major leg arteries (15). The ABI typically reported in published clinical studies is not obtained with an automated blood pressure cuff but rather with a sphygmomanometer or other medical-grade blood pressure device, and systolic pressure is determined with the help of a Doppler device. But the home-style test is valuable nevertheless, because it is usually good enough to alert one to seek medical consultation.

In 2009, *Archives of Cardiovascular Diseases* reported a study titled "Accuracy of ankle-brachial index using an automatic blood pressure device to detect peripheral artery disease in preventive medicine." The authors concluded that the correlations between the automatic and Doppler methods were good in left and right legs even in patients with an abnormal automatic index. The automatic method had good sensitivity (92%), specificity (98%), positive predictive value (86%), negative predictive value (99%) and accuracy (97%) compared with the Doppler method (16).

Cardiovascular and Sensory, Motor and Cognitive Disorders

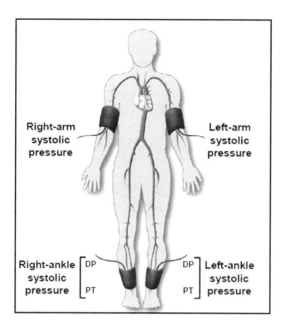

FIGURE 5.2 Cuff placement over the right, left (arm) brachial artery, and over the right, left (leg) anterior tibial artery. Source: https://www.ncbi.nlm.nih.gov/projects/gap/cgi-bin/document.cgi?study_id=phs000888.v1.p1&phd=4993

TABLE 5.1
Based on Measuring and Understanding the Ankle-Brachial Index (ABI)

ABI Value	Interpretation	Recommendation
Greater than 1.4	Calcification/Vessel Hardening	Refer to vascular specialist
1.0–1.4	Normal None 0.9–1.0 Acceptable	None
0.8–0.9	Some Arterial Disease	Treat risk factors
0.5–0.8	Moderate Arterial Disease	Refer to vascular specialist
Less than 0.5	Severe Arterial Disease	Refer to vascular specialist

Source: https://stanfordmedicine25.stanford.edu/the25/ankle-brachial-index.html; accessed June 10, 2022.

There may be some concerns about the trustworthiness of the index in certain clinical conditions where, for instance, there may be significant hardening of the arteries and in some cases, in diabetes. But they do not detract from the present message that ABI has been shown to be a useful index of the severity of conditions that impair endothelial function. So, anyone can try this at home.

5.4 THE ABI AND ENDOTHELIAL DYSFUNCTION

According to a 2003 report in the *Journal of Vascular Surgery*, the ABI, when adjusted for age, gender and classic cardiovascular risk factors, strongly indicates endothelial dysfunction (17).

The lower the ABI, the greater the risk of heart disease. A 1992 study titled "Ankle-arm index as a marker of atherosclerosis in the Cardiovascular Health Study" was conducted by the Cardiovascular Heart Study (CHS) Collaborative Research Group and published in the journal of the AHA, *Circulation*. An inverse relationship was found between the ABI (here labeled "ankle-arm index") and the cardiovascular risk factors and evidence of cardiovascular disease (CVD) in older adults. However, it was also the case that even those with no symptoms but a modest reduction in the ABI (0.8 to 1.0) appear to be at increased risk of PAD, heart and kidney disease (18).

5.5 OMEGA-3 FATTY ACID DEFICIENCY IN PERIPHERAL ARTERY DISEASE

A clinical study published in the journal *Lipids*, in 2019, reported that patients with PAD had a significantly lower mean Omega-3 Index. An absolute decrease of 1% in the Omega-3 Index was associated with 39% greater risk of developing PAD. Therefore, the investigators concluded that deficiency of omega-3 FAs is a feature of PAD (19).

So, there's a good way to find out if body omega-3 FAs are low, because the lower they are, the lower will be the ABI. And here is why one might consider trying this at home. A study published in the *Journal of the American Medical Association* (JAMA) in 2008, concluded that the ABI yields a more accurate prediction of cardiovascular risk than the conventional Framingham Risk Score (FRS) (20). And what's best is that where circulation in the limbs is marginal to poor, the ABI shows improvement with supplementation of omega-3 FAs.

5.5.1 THE HIGHER BODY OMEGA-3 FATTY ACIDS, THE HIGHER THE ABI

A study published in 2019 in the journal *Nutrition and Dietetics* aimed to determine whether dietary intake of omega-3 FAs would show up in risk indicators such as the ABI in a group of overweight and obese participants volunteering for a weight loss trial. It was found that, among other things, higher intake of omega-3 FAs was significantly associated with a higher ABI (21). A higher intake of omega-3s makes the ABI even higher, and that is GOOD.

Other previous investigations had also found that omega-3 FA supplementation, fish consumption, older age and smoking history affect the Omega-3 Index in different patient populations, although similar correlations have never been explored in PAD.

Prior fish oil supplementation predicts a higher Omega-3 Index. Smoking lowers it. A study published in the *Journal of Vascular Surgery*, in 2014, aimed to determine whether blood content of omega-3 FAs would directly and positively correlate with a history of fish oil supplementation and older age and inversely correlate with a smoking history and obesity. It was found that in patients with PAD, older age, elevated body mass index and prior fish oil supplementation predicted a higher Omega-3 Index. Smokers have a lower Omega-3 Index (22). Smoking-induced oxidative stress lowers levels of omega-3 FAs in plasma and brain tissue (23).

5.6 OSTEO- AND RHEUMATOID ARTHRITIS

Osteoarthritis, the most common form of arthritis, involves the loss of the cartilage that caps the bones in our joints. Rheumatoid arthritis is a disease where the immune system attacks the joints, beginning with the lining of joints. Both involve inflammation.

According to a 2016 report in the journal *Medical Hypotheses*, osteoarthritic pain indicates worsening endothelial function (24). And a 2003 report in the journal *Atherosclerosis* concludes that long-term rheumatoid arthritis is associated with manifested endothelial dysfunction (25).

Fish oil lowers osteoarthritis specific pain. "Fish oil supplementation reduces osteoarthritis-specific pain in older adults with overweight/obesity" was the title of a study published in 2020 in the journal *Rheumatology. Advances in Practice*. Sedentary overweight/obese older adults were given 2,000 milligrams (mg)/day docosahexaenoic acid (DHA) + 400 mg/day eicosapentaenoic (EPA) acid, 160 mg/day of curcumin or a combination of both for 16 weeks. Fish oil significantly reduced osteoarthritis specific pain compared to no fish oil treatment. Pain reduction was accompanied by improvements in small blood vessel function and well-being. Curcumin, alone or in combination with fish oil, did not reduce pain measures (26). However, a systematic review of research and clinical reports on the effects of curcumin titled "Curcumin: A review of its effects on human health," published in the journal *Foods*, in 2017, concludes that it has been shown to be very effective in reducing pain especially when its bioavailability is increased with piperine (by up to 2,000%) (27).

However, in one study, high dosage vs low dosage of omega-3s resulted in a paradoxical finding: In 2016, the journal *Annals of the Rheumatic Diseases* reported a clinical study where patients with knee osteoarthritis (OA) received either 4.5 grams (g) (high-dose), or 0.45 g (low dose) of omega-3 FAs for 24 months. The surprising finding was in the pain outcomes. As is frequent in OA trials, pain diminished in both groups, but it decreased more in the group on low-dose fish oil at 18 and 24 months for both pain and function. The investigators could not explain this seeming paradox (28). In any event, it was concluded that in people with symptomatic knee OA, there is no additional benefit of high-dose fish oil compared with low-dose fish oil. Not on knee joint pain anyway. But the higher dose did reduce triglycerides.

Fish oil decreases the number of tender joints and shortens the duration of morning stiffness in rheumatoid arthritis. A meta-analysis pools the findings of single independent studies using statistical methods to calculate an overall or "absolute effect." A meta-analysis published in the *Journal of Clinical Epidemiology*, in 1995, concluded that dietary fish oil supplementation for 3 months significantly reduced tender joint and morning stiffness compared to dietary control oils (29).

Omega-3 FAs at dosages greater than 2.7 g/day for more than 3 months reduces need for non-steroidal anti-inflammatory drugs (NSAIDs) by rheumatoid arthritis patients. Another meta-analysis published in the journal *Archives of Medical Research*, in 2012, aimed to determine the effects of ca. 2.7 g/day omega-3 FAs over a period of at least 3 months on clinical outcomes in patients with rheumatoid arthritis. It was found that omega-3 FAs significantly reduced the need for NSAIDs (30).

By the way, one teaspoon of fish oil weighs ca 4.50 g. We can calculate any dosage of fish oil by the teaspoon at https://www.traditionaloven.com/foods/exchange/tsp/g-gram/fish-oil-cod-liver.html.

5.7 OMEGA-3 FATTY ACIDS IMPROVE FILTRATION IN CHRONIC KIDNEY DISEASE

One in three American adults is at risk of kidney disease. In chronic kidney disease (CKD), the kidneys are damaged and can't properly filter blood. The main risk factors for developing kidney disease are diabetes, high blood pressure, heart disease and a family history of kidney failure. The National Kidney Foundation encourages us to "know your numbers." As noted in a report in the journal *Comprehensive Physiology* in 2013, chronic and acute renal diseases, irrespective of the initiating cause, have inflammation and immune system activation as a common underlying mechanism. The title of that report is "Immune and inflammatory role in renal disease" (31).

We need to be concerned with two kidney "numbers," the albumin-creatinine ratio (ACR) and the glomerular filtration rate (GFR). These numbers can be found on the routine medical blood and urine tests, the tests that physicians order with each medical checkup. GFR will determine what stage of kidney disease one may have. There are five of them. ACR is a urine test to see how much of a type of protein (albumin) there is in urine. Excess urine albumin is an early sign of kidney damage.

Having protein in urine may mean that the kidneys are not adequately filtering the blood. This can be a sign of early kidney disease. Three positive results over 3 months or more is a sign of kidney disease. When the kidneys are damaged, they have difficulty removing a waste product, creatinine, from the blood.

Everyone has creatinine in their bloodstream. It is a waste product that comes from the normal wear and tear of muscles of the body. Healthy kidneys filter creatinine out of the blood into the urine. Creatinine clearance (CrCl) is the volume of blood cleared of creatinine per unit of time. It is a test used to estimate the GFR. Testing for creatinine is only the first step, then the creatinine level is used to calculate the GFR, a number that reveals how well the kidneys are working (32) (Table 5.2).

There are two broad categories of kidney disease: Chronic kidney disease (CKD), longstanding disease of the kidneys leading to renal failure; and acute renal failure, a condition where the kidneys suddenly can't filter waste from the blood.

Most of the time, a GFR of 90 or more means the kidneys are healthy and working well. ACR levels (ratios) between 30–300 mg/g (category A2), indicate moderately increased albuminuria levels, a sign of early kidney disease. ACR levels greater

TABLE 5.2
Criteria for Severity of GFR as an Indication of Kidney Failure

GFR Category	GFR (mL/min/1.73 m^2)	Terms
G1	≥90	Normal or high
G2	60–89	Mildly decreased
G3a	45–59	Mildly to moderately decreased
G3b	30–44	Moderately to severely decreased
G4	15–29	Severely decreased
G5	<15	Kidney failure

Source: Based on 2013. KDIGO 2012 Clinical Practice Guideline for the Evaluation and Management of Chronic Kidney Disease. *Kidney International Supplements*, Jan; 3(1): 1–150. https://kdigo.org/wp-content/uploads/2017/02/KDIGO_2012_CKD_GL.pdf.

than 300 mg/g (category A3), indicate severely increased albuminuria levels, a sign of severe kidney disease. It is important to keep these numbers in mind because the outcome of omega-3 supplementation should show up as desirable changes in those numbers.

Endothelial dysfunction occurs in CKD and raises the risk for cardiovascular disease. The mechanisms of endothelial dysfunction seem to stem from impaired nitric oxide bioavailability (33).

Unlike some other medical disorders in which it has been reported, there is nothing in published medical reports that indicates that kidney failure may be due to omega-3 FA deficiency *per se*, but a number of clinical studies report the benefits of supplementation thereof. Such supplementation has been associated with a significantly reduced risk of end-stage renal disease and delays the progression of this disease. In fact, a higher Omega-3 Index was significantly associated with lower ACR in a young and healthy population with normal GFR. According to a 2021 report in the journal *Frontiers in Cardiovascular Medicine*, omega-3 FAs may actually be heart and kidney protective in healthy persons (34).

Older adults with low total plasma omega-3 FA levels have a greater decline in creatinine clearance (which is bad). A meta-analysis published in 2017, in the journal *Clinics* (Sao Paulo), reported that any or high-dose omega-3 FA supplementation, respectively, was associated with a lower risk of elevated albumin in urea with a significantly reduced risk of end-stage kidney disease and delay of the progression of this disease (35). This study showed that older adults with low total plasma FA levels have a greater decline in creatinine clearance over 3 years of follow-up. These findings suggest that a higher dietary intake of omega-3 FAs may be protective against progression to chronic kidney disease.

Protein energy wasting (PEW) is a state of decreased body stores of protein and energy fuels, and is associated with diminished functional capacity, impaired quality of life and increased mortality in patients with CKD. The prevalence of PEW ranges from 30 to 70% among patients on maintenance hemodialysis.

5.7.1 OMEGA-3S FROM FISH OIL IMPROVE QUALITY OF LIFE IN DIALYSIS PATIENTS

A clinical study published in the journal *Food and Nutrition Research*, in 2020, reported that fish oil intake in patients undergoing hemodialysis can significantly reduce PEW, and improve the quality of life of patients undergoing dialysis (36).

5.8 IRRITABLE BOWEL SYNDROME (IBS)

According to the Mayo Clinic, Irritable Bowel Syndrome (IBS) can develop after a severe bout of gastroenteritis caused by bacteria or a virus, or a surplus of bacteria in the intestines (bacterial overgrowth), or early life stress (37). More likely, according to a 2014 report in the journal *Pathogens*, it is due to infection by the bacteria, *Mycobacterium avium* subspecies *paratuberculosis* (38). And it can apparently be successfully treated with antibiotics (39).

According to a 2016 report in the *World Journal of Gastroenterology*, endothelial dysfunction is considered one of the causal factors of inflammatory bowel disease (IBD). The inflammation leads to impairment of the endothelium (40). Leaving aside cause, for the moment, it is an inflammatory condition and omega-3 FAs have been demonstrably beneficial in relieving inflammation, in general. As we are about to see, these FAs will also relieve IBS to an extent.

Women with IBS were found to have lower DHA and total omega-3 FA blood levels than a comparable group free of IBS. Interestingly, there is a rise in the incidence of IBS in Asia, especially among women. The investigators, in a study published in 2017 in the journal *Medicine*, thought that it might be due to deficiency in essential FAs due to malnutrition. They compared the nutritional status of a group of Asian women with IBS to that of a "healthy control" group. They found higher plasma saturated FAs and monounsaturated FAs, and lower DHA and total omega-3 FAs in the blood of the women with IBS (41).

Another study, published in 2014 in the *Journal of Crohn's and Colitis*, sought to determine whether inflammation of the colon would alter the bioavailability of the eicosanoid precursors arachidonic acid (AA), an omega-6 FA, and EPA, an omega-3 FA. It was found that biopsy samples collected from ulcerative colitis (UC) patients (vs non-UC controls) had significantly higher AA and significantly lower EPA contents and a significantly higher AA:EPA ratio. The AA:EPA ratio is, of course, the omega-6:omega-3 ratio. Furthermore, higher AA, AA:EPA ratio, DPA and DHA and lower LA, alpha-LNA and EPA as seen in inflamed mucosa in UC correlate with severity of inflammation, suggesting an alteration in FA metabolism in the inflamed gut mucosa in this disorder (42).

A review published in the journal *Annals of Gastroenterology* in 2016 reported that, although there is some controversy regarding the effects of omega-3 FAs in the prevention or treatment of IBD, their effects in reducing inflammation and pain are incontestable (43). That report cited intriguing work on an important aspect of pain control namely that DHA appears to reduce pain indirectly through the release of the endogenous opioid peptide β-endorphin, and not only because it acts on the opioid receptor (44). Other studies cited showed that increased consumption of omega-3 FAs and decreased consumption of omega-6 FAs can reduce pain through endocannabinoid* production (45).

IBS, and the controversy regarding its cause aside, is an inflammatory disease, yet a number of reviews and meta-analyses find no basis on which to recommend omega-3 FA supplementation. A reported omega-6:omega-3 ratio imbalance is equally curious and remains unexplained.

5.9 GLAUCOMA AND MACULAR DEGENERATION

Glaucoma is vision loss due to elevated fluid pressure inside the eye (intraocular) that damages the optic nerve. It can occur at any age, but it is one of the leading causes of blindness for people over the age of 60. Currently, the only known modifiable risk factor for glaucoma is intraocular fluid pressure. Many forms of glaucoma have no warning signs and the effect is so gradual that one may not notice a change in vision until the condition is at an advanced and irreversible stage.

A report in 2019 in the journal *Therapeutic Advances in Ophthalmology* concluded that there is an impairment of small blood vessel endothelial function and endothelial-independent blood flow regulation in primary open angle glaucoma (POAG) patients (46). The arterial blood vessels endothelium plays an important role in the regulation of blood flow in the eye and disease alterations of the endothelial cells may induce impaired blood flow observed in glaucoma.

Endothelial dysfunction in age-related macular degeneration (AMD) indicates subclinical atherosclerosis, according to a report in 2019 in the journal *Cutaneous and Ocular Toxicology* (47). And glaucoma patients have significantly reduced levels of EPA, DHA and total omega-3 FAs.

POAG, which is the commonest cause of non-remediable blindness and visual impairment, has no known cause. Increased intraocular pressure and blood vessel factors noted in this disorder are influenced by FAs. The purpose of a study published in 2006 in the journal *Prostaglandins, Leukotrienes and Essential Fatty Acids*, was to determine whether glaucoma patients have an abnormal blood FA composition. Compared to their healthy siblings, the glaucoma patients were found to have significantly reduced EPA, DHA and total omega-3 FAs in red cells and plasma, along with elevated triglycerides. These findings may be significant, since EPA and DHA could benefit impaired blood vessels and, therefore, blood flow in the eye (48).

Increasing omega-3s while controlling overall daily FAs may protect against glaucoma. A comprehensive study published in 2018 in the *Journal of the American Medical Association* (JAMA)—*Ophthalmology* reported finding that increased daily dietary consumption levels of the omega-3 FAs, EPA and DHA, were associated with

---

* The *endocannabinoid* system plays important roles in the body well beyond the process it's named for, which is interacting with cannabis, also known as marijuana.

lower likelihood of the nerve damage caused by glaucoma. However, consumption levels of total FAs in the higher quartiles were associated with a higher risk of glaucoma, which may have resulted from the far-too higher intakes of omega-6 FAs as compared to omega-3 FAs. In fact, the odds of having glaucoma were nearly three times as high in participants whose daily dietary total FA consumption level was in the second and third quartiles compared with those whose intake was in the first quartile. The authors concluded that increasing the proportion of dietary omega-3s consumption while limiting overall daily FA intake may protect against glaucoma (49).

Oral omega-3 supplementation for 3 months significantly reduced intraocular eye pressure (IOP) in normotensive adults. A clinical study published in 2018 in the journal *Translational Vision Science and Technology* aimed to determine the efficacy and safety of oral omega-3 supplementation for treating ocular surface inflammation. For 90 days, adults in the treatment group with normal intraocular eye pressure (IOP less than <21 millimeters of mercury (mm Hg)), and without a current or prior glaucoma diagnosis, received an oral ca. 1,000 mg/day of EPA + ~500 mg/day DHA ± 900 mg/day alpha-linolenic acid supplement whereas a placebo group was given 1,500 mg/day supplement of olive oil. At day 90, IOP was significantly reduced in the omega-3 group; the controls saw a slight IOP increase. The investigators concluded that omega-3 supplementation for 3 months significantly reduced IOP in normotensive adults. And, to their knowledge, this is the first study to report that omega-3 FAs lower IOP in humans (50).

Finally, in a clinical study published in 2011 in the *International Journal of Ophthalmology*, it is reported that omega-3 FAs from cod liver oil—a combination of vitamin A and omega-3 FAs—are beneficial for glaucoma patients as they decrease IOP, increase ocular blood flow and improve optic nerve function. "In this article, we propose that cod liver oil, as a combination of vitamin A and omega-3 fatty acids, should be beneficial for the treatment of glaucoma" (51).

5.9.1 A Paradox

A study published in the *American Journal of Clinical Nutrition* in 2004 reported seemingly paradoxically that a high ratio of omega-6 to omega-3 polyunsaturated FAs appears to *increase* the risk of POAG, particularly high-tension POAG. This finding should be noted but it is not consistent with other reports concerning the 6:3 ratio and glaucoma (52).

Another study, published in 2014 in the journal *Clinical Nutrition* (Edinburgh, Scotland), aimed to determine whether there is a relationship between intake of omega-3 and omega-6 FAs and their ratio, and the incidence of glaucoma in participants aged 40 years or older at baseline. After a median follow-up time of 8.2 years, participants in the highest quintile of omega-6:3 ratio intake (lower omega-6 amounts) had a significantly higher risk of glaucoma than participants in the lowest quintile. The association was stronger in participants 40 years old or older (53). However, many websites available to consumers recommend FA supplementation for glaucoma. For instance:

- *Omega-3 May Reduce Glaucoma Risk*: https://www.optometry.org.au/workplace/omega-3-may-reduce-glaucoma-risk; accessed April 14, 2022.

- *Omega-3 FAs*: https://www.eyephysiciansoflongbeach.com/dry-eye-center-of-excellence/omega-3-fatty-acids/; accessed April 13, 2022.
- *Fish Oil Supplementation Helps Lower the Risk of Glaucoma and Ocular Hypertension*: https://blog.designsforhealth.com/node/804; accessed April 13, 2022.
- *Omega-3—The Key to Glaucoma*: https://www.htc.co.uk/post/omega3-the-key-to-glaucoma; accessed April 14, 2022.

Caveat: Despite some clearly positive reports, and considering the noted paradox, we would be inclined, until further evidence emerges, to be cautious about omega-3 FA supplementation in the case of glaucoma.

The retina is the back surface of the eye where all the cells that give rise to vision are located. It has three different functional layers. The outermost layer is the photoreceptor layer, made up of *rod* and *cone* cells that transform light projected on it into electric signals that are processed and then sent to the brain. It is in the center of the retina, the macula, where detailed vision occurs.

Macular degeneration causes vision loss in the center of the field of vision. In dry macular degeneration, the center of the retina deteriorates, whereas in wet macular degeneration, leaky blood vessels grow under the retina. Macular degeneration causes blurred vision. A number of clinical reports attest to the benefits of omega-3 FA supplementation in halting the progression of the disease.

In 2020, the journal *Nutrients* reported an interesting anonymous online survey of Australian and New Zealander optometrists' attitudes and self-reported practice in connection with omega-3 FAs for eye health, and their knowledge and understanding of potential risks and benefits. Questions included practitioner demographics and practice modality; self-reported practices and recommendations relating to diet, nutritional supplements and omega-3 FAs for AMD and dry eye disease (DED); and practitioner knowledge about omega-3 FAs.

Most respondents indicated recommending to their patients that they consume omega-3 FAs to improve their eye health. Sixty-eight percent of respondents indicated recommending omega-3-rich foods for AMD management, while 62% indicated recommending omega-3 supplements. Most respondents (78%) indicated recommending omega-3-rich foods or supplements for DED. For DED, recommended omega-3 supplement dosages were (median [inter-quartile range, IQR]) 2,000 mg (1,000–2,750 mg) per day. The main sources of information reported by respondents to guide their clinical decision making were continuing education articles and conferences (54).

Women who eat fish high in omega-3 FAs at least twice a week are less likely to develop AMD. The website of the American Academy of Ophthalmology (AAO) featured an article, "The benefits of fish oil for dry eye" (55). On another webpage, the AAO featured "Fish can lower AMD risk. Studies found that women who ate fish high in omega-3 fatty acids at least twice a week were less likely to get age-related macular degeneration (AMD)" (56). And the Harvard Health website featured "Omega-3 for your eyes. Research finds DHA may help preserve your vision."

5.10 OMEGA-3 FATTY ACID DHA PROTECTS VISION

A new study published in *Investigative Ophthalmology & Visual Science* found that DHA, one of three forms of omega-3 FAs and the substance that makes up about 30% of brain matter, prevented age-related vision loss in lab mice (57).

Fish consumption and progression of AMD—a clinical study published in the journal *Archives of Ophthalmology* in 2003 reported that among individuals with the early or intermediate stages of AMD, fish intake and nuts reduced risk (58). Fish and nuts, i.e., omega-3 and -6—it was also reported in the same journal in 2006, in a study on twins that cigarette smoking increases risk of AMD, while fish consumption and omega-3 FA supplement intake reduces the risk (59).

High intake of dietary omega-3 FAs or fish is associated with a reduced risk of developing AMD. Finally, a recent meta-analysis published in the journal *Clinical Nutrition* in 2021 reported that a dose-response analysis showed a 6% and 22% decrease in the risk of early and late AMD for each additional 1 g/day of omega-3 FA intake. For individual omega-3 FAs, the intake of EPA and DHA was inversely associated with lower AMD risk, whereas no association was found for alpha-linolenic acid.*

Consistent inverse associations were also found between fish intake and AMD. Every 15 g/day of fish consumption was associated with 13% and 14% lower early and late AMD. In addition, fish intake was associated with a significantly reduced risk of AMD progression. The authors concluded that a high intake of dietary omega-3 FAs, as supplements or as consumption of fish, is associated with a reduced risk of developing AMD, and they recommend consumption of omega-3 FA-rich foods as a new nutritional approach to preventing AMD (60).

5.11 BRAIN FISH OIL-LUBE FOR MILD COGNITIVE IMPAIRMENT IN AGING

Cognitive dysfunction refers to deficits in attention, verbal and nonverbal learning, short-term and working memory, visual and auditory processing, problem solving and processing speed. This condition is basically a mental disorder, and we will rather address here the expected cognitive decline of normal aging. In other words, the focus is on enhancing function, rather than correcting a mental disorder.

5.11.1 INFLAMM-AGING

The term "inflamm-aging" was coined by Franceschi, Bonafe, Valensin et al. in 2000, and it appeared in the title of their report, "Inflamm-aging: an evolutionary perspective on immunosenescence," in the *Annals of the New York Academy of Science*. The investigators contend that inflammation plays an important role in the rate of aging and age-related diseases (61). Inflammation leads to endothelium dysfunction. With advancing age, there are changes that occur in the blood vessels,

---

* Alpha-linolenic acid is a type of omega-3 FA found in plants. This suggests that fish beats flax for reducing risk and/or severity of AMD.

especially endothelial dysfunction, that affect how we process information, store it in memory, and how we think (61).

The Healthline website features an article titled "How omega-3 fish oil affects your brain and mental health." It tells us that omega-3s are vital for normal brain function and development and that low levels of omega-3s may accelerate brain aging and contribute to deficits in brain function. It cites studies that show that fish oil may benefit mild memory loss and that fish oil may lessen depression, a not uncommon feature in the aging (62).

In a clinical study published in the journal *Neurology* in 2012, investigators reported examining the relationship between red blood cell FA levels (read: Omega-3 Index) to brain markers of risk of cognitive dysfunction in a middle-aged to elderly community-based cohort. They found that participants with red blood cell DHA levels in the lowest quartile (Q1) when compared to others (Q2–Q4) had significantly lower total brain volumes (low brain volume being a sign of dementia). Participants with lower DHA and Omega-3 Index also had significantly lower scores on tests of visual memory, executive function and abstract thinking.

The investigators concluded that a lower Omega-3 Index is associated with smaller brain volumes and a "vascular" pattern of cognitive impairment even in persons free of clinical dementia. Notably, the Magnetic Resonance Imaging (MRI) finding of lower brain volume represents a change equivalent to approximately 2 years of structural brain aging (63).

Omega-3 supplementation has a positive effect on cognitive function in aged or elder adults. A systematic review of clinical studies titled "Omega-3 fatty acids and cognitive decline" was published in 2019 in the journal *Nutrición Hospitalaria*. The aim of the review was to determine the relationship between omega-3 FAs and cognitive status in aged adult and elder populations and to determine whether there is a beneficial effect of omega-3 FA supplementation on cognitive decline.

In that systematic review, a search of randomized controlled trials (RCTs) was conducted through PubMed database from January 2010 to December 2017. It was found that ten out of the 14 studies reviewed showed positive outcome on at least one domain of cognitive function (working memory, executive function, verbal memory, short-term memory, perceptual speed, etc.). The authors concluded that omega-3 supplementation has a positive effect on cognitive function and that it could be used as a preventive or therapeutic tool for cognitive decline in aged or elder adults (64).

Intake of omega-3 FAs has been shown to protect against mild cognitive impairment (MCI). The aim of a study published in 2017 in the journal *Nutrients* was to determine the effect of omega-3 FA supplementation on cognitive function in the Chinese elderly with MCI. Participants aged 60 years or older (mean age 71) were given either 480 mg DHA and 720 mg EPA per day of omega-3 FAs, or olive oil placebo. It was found that omega-3 FAs significantly improved total Basic Cognitive Aptitude Tests (BCAT) scores, perceptual speed, space imagery efficiency and working memory, but not mental arithmetic efficiency or recognition memory.

Subgroup analysis by gender showed that in men, omega-3 FAs significantly improved perceptual speed, space imagery efficiency, working memory and total BCAT scores. In women, the significant beneficial effects were observed in perceptual speed, space imagery efficiency and total BCAT scores, but not in working memory. The investigators concluded that omega-3 FAs can improve cognitive function in people with MCI (65).

It is not generally known that inflammation underlies all the above conditions and that what inflammation does is that it impairs endothelium function and that endothelial dysfunction, in turn, impairs blood flow to all parts of the body and that can spell disaster. So, by neglecting to support the endothelium with the antioxidants in omega-3 FAs, we encourage inflammation and there is a plethora of really nasty conditions that one can get from that neglect. However, with omega-3 FAs, we can prevent, even turn around accelerated cognitive decline. Here is what the experts say.

A recent (2020) clinical study published in the journal *Nutrients* aimed to determine the effects of a high-dose omega-3 and omega-6 FA supplementation in combination with antioxidant vitamins on cognitive function and functional capacity of older adults with MCI. For 6 months, the participants, 78.8 ± 7.3 years old, received either a 20 milliliter (mL) dose of a formula containing a mixture of omega-3 (810 mg EPA and 4,140 mg DHA) and omega-6 FAs (1,800 mg gamma-linolenic acid and 3,150 mg linoleic acid), with 0.6 mg vitamin A, vitamin E (22 mg) plus pure γ-tocopherol (760 mg) or 20 mL placebo containing olive oil.

A significant beneficial effect of supplementation was found on cognitive function, Mini-Mental State Examination, and Stroop Color and Word Test. Also, functional capacity consisting of a 6-minute walk test and sit-to-stand-60 test, examining fatigue, physical health and daily sleepiness, showed a favorable improvement for the participants receiving the supplement vs placebo. The investigators contend that these supplements could be promising for reducing cognitive and functional decline in the elderly with MCI (66).

REFERENCES

1. Dinh QN, Drummond GR, Sobey CG, and S Chrissobolis. 2014. Roles of inflammation, oxidative stress, and vascular dysfunction in hypertension. *BioMed Research International*, 14:ID 406960. DOI: 10.1155/2014/406960.
2. Conti P, and Y Shaik-Dasthagirisaeb. 2015. Atherosclerosis: A chronic inflammatory disease mediated by mast cells. *Central European Journal of Immunology*, 40(3): 380–386. DOI: 10.5114/ceji.2015.54603.
3. Christodoulidis GC, Vittorio TJ, Fudim M, Lerakis S, and CE Kosmas. 2014. Inflammation in coronary artery disease. *Cardiology in Review*, Nov/Dec; 22(6): 279–288. DOI: 10.1097/CRD.0000000000000006.
4. Tsalamandris S, Antonopoulos AS, Oikonomou E, Papamikroulis G-A, Vogiatzi G, Papaioannou S, Deftereos S, and D Tousoulis. 2019. The role of iflammation in diabetes: Current concepts and future perspectives. *European Cardiology*, Apr; 14(1): 50–59. DOI: 10.15420/ecr.2018.33.1.
5. Rapa SF, Di Iorio BR, Campiglia P, Heidland A, and S Marzocco. 2020. Inflammation and oxidative stress in chronic kidney disease—Potential therapeutic role of minerals, vitamins and plant-derived metabolites. *International Journal of Molecular Sciences, Jan*; 21(1): 263. DOI: 10.3390/ijms21010263.
6. Brevetti G, Giugliano G, Brevetti L, and WR Hiatt. 2010. Inflammation in peripheral artery disease. *Circulation*, 122: 1862–1875. DOI: https://doi.org/10.1161/CIRCULATIONAHA.109.918417.

7. https://health. ucsd.edu/news/releases/ pages/2014-07-14-acute-close-angle-glau coma .aspx; accessed 2/10/22)
8. Klein R, Myers CE, Cruickshanks KJ, Ronald E. Gangnon RE, Danforth LG, Sivakumaran TA, Iyengar SK, Tsai MY, and BEK Klein. 2014. Markers of inflammation, oxidative stress, and endothelial dysfunction and the 20-year cumulative incidence of early age-related macular degeneration. The Beaver Dam Eye Study. *JAMA Ophthalmology*, 132(4): 446–455. DOI: 10.1001/jamaophthalmol. 2013.7671.
9. Kumar A. 2018. Editorial: Neuroinflammation and cognition. *Frontiers in Aging Neuroscience*, 10: 413. DOI: 10.3389/fnagi.2018.00413.
10. Silvestro A, Oliva G, and G Brevetti. 2002. Intermittent claudication and endothelial dysfunction. *European Heart Journal Supplements*, 4(Supplement B): B35–B40.
11. https://www.heart.org/en/health-topics/peripheral-artery-disease/about-peripheral-artery-disease-pad; accessed 2/9/22.
12. Gerhard-Herman MD, Gornik HL, Barrett C, Barshes NR, Corriere MA, Drachman DE, Fleisher LA, Fowkes FGR, Hamburg NM, Kinlay S, Lookstein R, Misra S, Mureebe L, Olin JW, Patel RAG, Regensteiner JG, Schanzer A, Shishehbor MH, Stewart KJ, Treat-Jacobson D, and ME Walsh. 2017. 2016 AHA/ACC guideline on the management of patients with lower extremity peripheral artery disease: Executive summary: A Report of the American College of Cardiology/American Heart Association Task Force on Clinical Practice Guidelines. *Circulation*, 135(12): e686–e725. https://doi.org/10.1161/CIR.0000000000000470.
13. Fried R. 2014. *Erectile dysfunction as a cardiovascular impairment*. Academic Press/Elsevier Science.
14. McDermott MM, Criqui MH, Liu K, Guralnik JM, Greenland P, Martin GJ, and W Pearce. 2000. Lower ankle/brachial index, as calculated by averaging the dorsalis pedis and posterior tibial arterial pressures, and association with leg functioning in peripheral arterial disease. *Journal of Vascular Surgery*, 32, 1164–1171. DOI: 10.1067/mva.2000.108640.
15. Bernstein EF, and A Fronek. 1982. Current status of non-invasive tests in the diagnosis of peripheral arterial disease. *Surgical Clinics of North America*, 62, 473–487.
16. Benchimol D, Pillois X, Benchimol A, Houitte A, Sagardiluz P, Tortelier L, and J Bonnet. 2009. Détection de l'artériopathie des membres inférieurs en médecine préventive par la détermination de l'index de pression systolique à l'aide d'un tensiomètre automatique [Accuracy of ankle-brachial index using an automatic blood pressure device to detect peripheral artery disease in preventive medicine]. *Archives of Cardiovascular Diseases*, 102, 519–524.
17. Brevetti G, Silvestro A, Di Giacomo S, Di Donato AM, Schiano V, and F Scopacasa. 2003. Endothelial dysfunction in peripheral arterial disease is related to increase in plasma markers of inflammation and severity of peripheral circulatory impairment but not to classic risk factors and atherosclerotic burden. *Journal of Vascular Surgery*, Aug 1; 38(2): P374–379. DOI: 10.1016/S0741-5214(03)00124-1.
18. Newman AB, Siscovick DS, Manolio TA, Polak J, Fried LP, Borhani NO, and SK Wolfson. 1993. Ankle-arm index as a marker of atherosclerosis in the Cardiovascular Health Study. Cardiovascular Heart Study (CHS) Collaborative Research Group. *Circulation*, 88, 837–845. DOI: 10.1161/01.CIR.88.3.837.
19. Ramirez JL, Zahner GJ, Spaulding KA, Khetani SA, Hills NK, Gasper WJ, Harris WS, Cohen BE, and SM Grenon. 2019. Peripheral artery disease is associated with a deficiency of erythrocyte membrane n-3 polyunsaturated fatty acids. *Lipids*, Apr; 54(4): 211–219. DOI: https://doi.org/10.1002/ lipd.12140.
20. Fowkes FG, Murray GD, Butcher I, Heald CL, Lee RJ, Chambless LE, Folsom AR, Hirsch AT, Dramaix M, deBacker G, Wautrecht JC, Kornitzer M, Newman

AB, Cushman M, Sutton-Tyrrell K, Fowkes FG, Lee AJ, Price JF, d'Agostino RB, Murabito JM, Norman PE, Jamrozik K, Curb JD, Masaki KH, Rodriguez BL, Dekker JM, Bouter LM, Heine RJ, Nijpels G, Stehouwer CD, Ferrucci L, McDermott MM, Stoffers HE, Hooi JD, Knottnerus JA, Ogren M, Hedblad B, Witteman JC, Breteler MM, Hunink MG, Hofman A, Criqui MH, Langer RD, Fronek A, Hiatt WR, Hamman R, Resnick HE, Guralnik J, McDermott MM. 2008. Ankle brachial index combined with Framingham Risk Score to predict cardiovascular events and mortality: a meta-analysis. *JAMA*, Jul 9; 300(2): 197–208. DOI: 10.1001/ jama.300.2.197.

21. Senevirathne A, Neale E, Peoples G, and L Tapsell. 2019. Relationship between long-chain omega-3 polyunsaturated fatty acid intake and ankle brachial index, pulse wave velocity and resting heart rate in a sample of overweight adults: A secondary analysis of baseline data in the HealthTrack study. *Nutrition and Dietetics*, Feb; 76(1): 95–103. DOI: 10.1111/1747-0080.12479.

22. Nosova EV, Chong KC, Alley HF, Conte MS, Owens CD, and SM Grenon. 2014. Clinical correlates of red blood cell omega-3 fatty acid content in male veterans with peripheral arterial disease. *Journal of Vascular Surgery*, 60(5): 1325–1331. DOI: https://doi.org/10.1016/j.jvs.2014.05.040.

23. Sadeghi-Ardekani K, Haghighi M, and R Zarrin. 2018. Effects of omega-3 fatty acid supplementation on cigarette craving and oxidative stress index in heavy-smoker males: A double-blind, randomized, placebo-controlled clinical trial. *Journal of Psychopharmacology*, Sep; 32(9): 995–1002. DOI: 10.1177/0269881118788806.

24. Laskarin G, Persic V, Rusac Kukic S, Massari D, Legovic A, Boban M, Miskulin R, Rogoznica M, and T Kehler. 2016. Can pain intensity in osteoarthritis joint be indicator of the impairment of endothelial function? *Medical Hypotheses*, Sep; 94:15–9. DOI: 10.1016/j.mehy.2016.06.001.

25. Hänsel S, Lässig G, Pistrosch F, and J Passauer. 2003. Endothelial dysfunction in young patients with long-term rheumatoid arthritis and low disease activity. *Atherosclerosis*, Sep 1; 170(1): 177–180. DOI: https://doi.org/10.1016/S0021-9150(03)00281-8.

26. Kuszewski JC, Wong RH, and PRC Hower. 2020. Fish oil supplementation reduces osteoarthritis-specific pain in older adults with overweight/obesity. *Rheumatology. Advances in Practice*. 4(2): rkaa036. DOI: 10.1093/rap/rkaa036.

27. Hewlings SJ, and DS Kalman. 2017. Curcumin: A review of its effects on human health. *Foods*, Oct; 6(10): 92. DOI: 10.3390/foods6100092.

28. Hill CL, March LM, Aitken D, Lester SE, Battersby R, Kristen Hynes K, Fedorova T, Proudman SM, James M, Cleland LG, and G Jones. 2016. Fish oil in knee osteoarthritis: a randomised clinical trial of low dose versus high dose. *Annals of the Rheumatic Diseases, Jan*; 75(1): 23–29. DOI: 10.1136/annrheumdis-2014-207169.

29. Fortin PR, Lew RA, Liang MH, Wright EA, Beckett LA, Chalmers TC, and RI Sperling. 1995. Validation of a meta-analysis: The effects of fish oil in rheumatoid arthritis. *Journal of Clinical Epidemiology*, Nov; 48(11): 1379–1390. DOI: 10.10 16/0895-4356(95)00028-3.

30. Lee Y-H, Bae S-C, and G-G Song. 2012. Omega-3 polyunsaturated fatty acids and the treatment of rheumatoid arthritis: A meta-analysis. *Archives of Medical Research*, Jul; 43(5): 356–362. DOI: 10.1016/j.arcmed.2012.06.011.

31. Imig JD, and MJ Ryan. 2013. Immune and inflammatory role in renal disease. *Comprehensive Physiology*, Apr; 3(2): 957–976. DOI: 10.1002/cphy.c120028.

32. https://www.kidney.org/atoz/content/know-your-kidney-numbers-two-simple-tests#:~:text=Know%20your%20kidney%20numbers!,have%20E2%80%93there%20are%205%20stages; accessed 2/13/22.

33. Martens CR, Kirkman DL, and DG Edwards. 2016. The vascular endothelium in chronic kidney disease: A novel target for aerobic exercise. *Exercise and Sport Sciences Review, Jan*; 44(1): 12–19. DOI: 10.1249/JES.0000000000000065.
34. Filipovic MG, Reiner MF, Rittirsch S, Irincheeva I, Aeschbacher S, Grossmann K, Risch M, Risch L, Limacher A, Conen D, and JH Beer. 2021. Blood omega-3 fatty acids are inversely associated with albumin-creatinine ratio in young and healthy adults (The Omega-Kid Study). *Frontiers in Cardiovascular Medicine*, 8: 622619. DOI: 10.3389/fcvm.2021.622619.
35. Hu J, Liu Z, and H Zhang. 2017. Omega-3 fatty acid supplementation as an adjunctive therapy in the treatment of chronic kidney disease: A meta-analysis. *Clinics (Sao Paulo), Jan*; 72(1): 58–64. DOI: 10.6061/clinics/2017(01)10.
36. Zhang C, Ge C, Wang, J, and D Sun. (2020. Effects of fish oil during hemodialysis on nutritional status and quality of life: a randomized double-blinded trial. *Food and Nutrition Research*, 64. https://doi.org/10.29219/fnr.v64.4450.
37. https://www.mayoclinic.org/diseases-conditions/irritable-bowel-syndrome/symptoms-causes/syc-20360016; accessed 2/15/22.
38. Rhodes G, Richardson H, Hermon-Taylor J, Weightman A, Higham A, and R Pickup. 2014. *Mycobacterium avium* subspecies *paratuberculosis*: Human exposure through environmental and domestic aerosols. *Pathogens, Sep*; 3(3): 577–595. DOI: 10. 3390/pathogens3030577.
39. Savarino E, Bertani L, Ceccarelli L, Bodini G, Zingone F, Buda A, Facchin S, Lorenzon G, Marchi S, Marabotto E, De Bortoli N, Savarino V, Costa F, and C Blandizzi. 2019. Antimicrobial treatment with the fixed-dose antibiotic combination RHB-104 for *Mycobacterium avium* subspecies *paratuberculosis* in Crohn's disease: Pharmacological and clinical implications. *Expert Opinion on Biological Therapy, Feb*; 19(2): 79–88. DOI: 10.1080/14712598.2019.1561852.
40. Cibor D, Domagala-Rodacka R, Rodacki T, Jurczyszyn A, Mach T, and D Owczarek. 2016. Endothelial dysfunction in inflammatory bowel diseases: Pathogenesis, assessment and implications. *World Journal of Gastroenterology, Jan* 21; 22(3): 1067–1077. DOI: 10.3748/wjg.v22.i3.1067.
41. Chua CS, Huang S-Y, Cheng C-W, Bai C-H, Hsu C-Y, Chiu H-W, and J-L Hsu. Fatty acid components in Asian female patients with irritable bowel syndrome. 2017. *Medicine*, Dec; 96(49): e9094. DOI: 10.1097/MD.0000000000009094.
42. Pearl DS, Masoodi M, Eiden M, Brümmer J, Gullick D, McKeever T, Whittaker MA, Nitch-Smith H, Brown JF, Shute JK, Mills G, Calder PC, and TM Trebble. 2014. Altered colonic mucosal availability of n-3 and n-6 polyunsaturated fatty acids in ulcerative colitis and the relationship to disease activity. *Journal of Crohn's and Colitis*, Jan; 8(1): 70–79. DOI: 10.1016/j.crohns.2013.03.013.
43. Barbalho SM, Goulart R de A, Quesada K, Bechara MD, and A de C Alves de Carvalhoe. 2016. Inflammatory bowel disease: can omega-3 fatty acids really help? *Annals of Gastroenterology*, Jan–Mar; 29(1); 37–43. PMCID: PMC4700845.
44. Nakamoto K, Nishinaka T, Ambo A, Mankura M, Kasuya F, and S Tokuyama. 2011. Possible involvement of β-endorphin in docosahexaenoic acid-induced antinociception. *European Journal of Pharmacology*, Sep; 666(1–3): 100–104. DOI: 10.1016/j.ejphar.2011.05.047.
45. Ramsden CE, Zamora D, Makriyannis A, Wood JA T, Mann JD, Faurot KR, MacIntosh BA, Majchrzak-Hong SF, Gross JR, Courville AB, Davis JM, and JR Hibbeln. 2015. Diet-induced changes in n-3- and n-6-derived endocannabinoids and reductions in headache pain and psychological distress. *Journal of Pain*, Aug; 16(8): 707–716. DOI: 10.1016/j.jpain.2015.04.007.

46. Bukhari SMI, Yew KK, Thambiraja R, Sulong S, Rasool AHG, and L-SA Tajudin. 2019. Microvascular endothelial function and primary open angle glaucoma. *Therapeutic Advances in Ophthalmology*, Jan–Dec; 11: 2515841419868100. DOI: 10.1177/ 2515841419868100.
47. Baltu F, Sarici AM, Yildirim O, Mergen B, and E Bolat. 2019. Investigation of vascular endothelial dysfunction in the patients with age-related macular degeneration. Mar; 38(1): 29–35. DOI: 10.1080/15569527.2018.1504056.
48. Ren H, Magulike N, Ghebremeskel K, and M Crawford. 2006. Primary open-angle glaucoma patients have reduced levels of blood docosahexaenoic and eicosapentaenoic acids. *Prostaglandins, Leukotrienes and Essential Fatty Acids*, Mar; 74(3): 157–163. DOI: 10.1016/j.plefa.2005.11.007.
49. Wang YE, Tseng VL, Yu F, Caprioli J, and AL Coleman. 2018. Association of dietary fatty acid intake with glaucoma in the United States. *JAMA Ophthalmology*, Feb; 136(2): 141–147. DOI:10.1001/jamaophthalmol.2017.5702.
50. Downie LE, and AJ Vingrys. 2018. Oral omega-3 supplementation lowers intraocular pressure in normotensive adults. *Translational Vision Science and Technology*, May; 7(3): 1. DOI: 10.1167/tvst.7.3.1.
51. Huang W-B, Fan Q, and X-L Zhang. 2011. Cod liver oil: A potential protective supplement for human glaucoma. *International Journal of Ophthalmology*, 4(6): 648–651. DOI: 10.3980/j.issn.2222-3959.2011.06.15.
52. Kang JH, Pasquale LR, Willett WC, Rosner BA, Egan KM, Faberowski N, and SE Hankinson. 2004. Dietary fat consumption and primary open-angle glaucoma. *American Journal of Clinical Nutrition*, May; 79(5): 755–764. DOI: 10.1093/ajcn/79.5.755.
53. Pérez de Arcelus M, Toledo E, Martínez-González MA, Sayón-Orea C, Gea A, and J Moreno-Montañés. 2014. Omega 3:6 ratio intake and incidence of glaucoma: The SUN cohort. *Clinical Nutrition (Edinburgh, Scotland)*, Dec; 33(6): 1041–1045. DOI: 10.1016/j.clnu.2013.11.005.
54. Zhang AC, Singh S, Craig JP, and LE Downie 2020. Omega-3 fatty acids and eye health: Opinions and self-reported practice behaviors of optometrists in Australia and New Zealand. *Nutrients*, Apr; 12(4): 1179. DOI: 10.3390/nu12041179.
55. https://www.aao.org/eye-health/tips-prevention/does-fish-oil-help-dry-eye#:~:text= Stephanie%20Marioneaux%2C%20MD%2C%20a%20spokesperson%20for%20the %20American,sense%20that%20a%20supplement%20could%20help%20the%20problem; accessed 2/17/22.
56. https://www.aao.org/eye-health/tips-prevention/diet-nutrition; accessed 2/17/22.
57. https://www. health.harvard.edu/heart-health/omega-3-for-your-eyes; accessed 2/17/22.
58. Seddon JM, Cote J, and B Rosner. 2003. Progression of age-related macular degeneration: Association with dietary fat, transunsaturated fat, nuts, and fish intake. *Archives of Ophthalmology*, Dec; 121(12): 1728–1737. DOI: 10.1001/archopht. 121.12.1728.
59. Seddon JM, George S, and B Rosner. 2006. Cigarette smoking, fish consumption, omega-3 fatty acid intake, and associations with age-related macular degeneration: The US Twin Study of Age-Related Macular Degeneration. *Archives of Ophthalmology*, Jul; 124(7): 995–1001. DOI: 10.1001/archopht.124.7.995.
60. Jiang H, Shi X, Fan Y, Wang D, Li B, Zhou J, Pei C, and L Ma. 2021. Dietary omega-3 polyunsaturated fatty acids and fish intake and risk of age-related macular degeneration. *Clinical Nutrition*, Dec; 40(12): 5662–5673. DOI: 10.1016/j.clnu. 2021.10.005.
61. Franceschi C, Bonafe M, Valensin S, Olivieri F, De Luca M, Ottaviani E and De Benedictis G (2000). "Inflamm-aging. An evolutionary perspective on immunosenescence." *Annals of the New York Academy of Sciences*, Jun; 908: 244–254. DOI: 10.1111/ j.1749-6632.2000.tb06651.x .

62. Fish Oil May Improve Depression; accessed 2/17/22.
63. Tan ZS, Harris WS, Beiser AS, Au R, Himali JJ, Debette S, Pikula A, DeCarli C, Wolf PA, Vasan RS, Robins SJ, and S Seshadri. 2012. Red blood cell omega-3 fatty acid levels and markers of accelerated brain aging. *Neurology*, Feb 28; 78(9): 658–664. DOI: 10.1212/WNL.0b013e318249f6a9.
64. Martí Del Moral A, and F Fortique. 2019. Omega-3 fatty acids and cognitive decline: a systematic review. *Nutrición Hospitalaria*, Aug 26; 36(4): 939–949. DOI: 10.20 960/nh.02496.
65. Bo Y, Zhang X, Wang Y, You J, Cui H, Zhu Y, Pang W, Liu W, Jiang Y, and Q Lu. 2017. The n-3 polyunsaturated fatty acids supplementation improved the cognitive function in the Chinese elderly with mild cognitive impairment: A double-blind randomized controlled trial. *Nutrients*, Jan 10; 9(1): 54. DOI: 10.3390/nu9010054.
66. Stavrinou PS, Andreou E, Aphamis G, Pantzaris M, Ioannou M, Patrikios IS, and CD Giannaki. 2020. The effects of a 6-month high dose omega-3 and omega-6 polyunsaturated fatty acids and antioxidant vitamins supplementation on cognitive function and functional capacity in older adults with mild cognitive impairment. *Nutrient*, Feb; 12(2): 325. DOI: 10.3390/nu12020325.

6 Flax I: A Pharaoh's Garment, a Roman's Laxative

> All that man needs for health and healing has been provided by God in nature, the challenge of science is to find it.
>
> —Paracelsus

6.1 THOSE BLUE FLOWER ROADSIDE WEEDS?

Driving down a country road, one often sees those little blue flowers growing like weeds. Most people pay scant attention to them. Yet their stalks had made garments for the Pharaohs, their seeds were laxatives for the Romans; until recently we made fine linen from flax, and today, we also use the oil to "finish" wood furniture. Cotton has pretty much replaced it as the major source of linen, but we've kept its name, linen, from *Linum usitatissimum* L. Parenthetically, *usitatissimum* means "most useful." Which it certainly is as it is also jam-packed with alpha-linolenic acid (ALA), a powerful antioxidant omega-3 fatty acid (FA) and lignans.

Lignans are steroid-like phytoestrogens, i.e., plant estrogens. They are found in plants, particularly in seeds, whole grains and vegetables. Flaxseed is the richest known source of lignans (9–30 milligrams/gram [mg/g]) (1). The principal dietary lignan in flaxseed is secoi-solari-ciresinol di-gluco-side (SDG) [hyphens added to facilitate pronunciation], an antioxidant phytoestrogen also presents in sunflower, sesame and pumpkin seeds. But flaxseed contains the highest total phytoestrogen content followed by soybean and tofu.

In many clinical studies on the effects of "flax," the lignans are extracted from the seeds and used as the treatment. For instance, a study published in 2016 in the journal *Current Pharmaceutical Design* reports slowing of progression (and even regression) of atherosclerosis with the flaxseed-derived lignans SDG (2).

Phytoestrogens are natural compounds found in plants and plant-based foods that imitate estrogen because their chemical structure is very similar to that of the estrogen that our body make. When we consume them, they may affect us in the same way as the estrogen we produce; however, their effects may be weaker.

Although not as popular today as it once was, flax still has many uses: It is cultivated for its seeds which can be ground into meal or turned into flaxseed oil, a nutrition supplement. Flaxseed oil, as linseed oil, is an ingredient in many wood-finishing products. Flax also holds many *micronutrient* constituents in addition to a balance of omega-6s and omega-3s, along with the lignans we mentioned above and that promote health. It is often suspected that deficiency of these micronutrients contributes much to the abundance of medical disorders that plague us now, such as hypertension, atherosclerosis, heart failure, chronic kidney disease, Type 2 diabetes and many more. These micronutrients are vitamins, minerals and other antioxidants needed for healthy living.

Micronutrients are ordinarily contained in common foods we consume, but unfortunately, many are routinely eliminated in the production of "processed foods" that now constitute much of our food consumption. There is a compelling need to replace these micronutrients by supplementation.

6.2 FLAX IS A "FUNCTIONAL FOOD"

Functional foods have a positive effect on health beyond basic nutrition. They are said to promote optimal health and help reduce the risk of disease. Functional foods differ from *nutraceuticals*, a broad umbrella term that is used to describe any products derived from food sources with medicinal benefits. A food that holds one or more nutraceuticals would be considered a functional food. Flax fits that to a "t." So, if flax is so good for us, exactly how much of it should we consume just to stay healthy? Here is what the experts say.

According to a report titled "Human requirement for N-3 polyunsaturated fatty acids," published in the journal *Poultry Science*, in 2000, current dietary recommendations for adults suggest a daily intake of 2.22 g (0.08 ounces [oz]) of ALA based on a 2,000-kilocalorie (kcal) diet (3). Since 1 tablespoon (tbsp) (7 g) of ground flaxseed contains 1.6 g of ALA, so that comes to more than one, and less than 2 tbsp. You can expect that body ALA levels will rise as soon as 2 weeks after the initiation of flaxseed supplementation (4). Likewise, the Mayo Clinic website tells readers that while there are no specific recommendations for flaxseed intake, nevertheless 1–2 tbsp a day is considered a healthy amount. One tablespoon of ground flaxseed yields 37 calories (cal) and contains 2 g of polyunsaturated fat (including the omega-3 FAs), 0.5 g of monounsaturated fat, and 2 g of dietary fiber (5).

On the MedicineNet website we learn that guidelines do not specify the daily recommended intake of flaxseed. However, it states that most experts agree that 1–2 tbsp of flaxseeds a day is good for health (6). And, according to the Healthline website, 1 tbsp (7 g) of ground flaxseed contains:

- Calories: 37.
- Carbs: 2 g.
- Fat: 3 g.
- Fiber: 2 g.
- Protein: 1.3 g.
- Thiamine: 10% of the Daily Value (DV).
- Copper: 9% of the DV.
- Manganese: 8% of the DV.

- Magnesium: 7% of the DV.
- Phosphorus: 4% of the DV.
- Selenium: 3% of the DV.
- Zinc: 3% of the DV.
- Vitamin B6: 2% of the DV.
- Iron: 2% of the DV.
- Folate: 2% of the DV.

Many of the health benefits noted in the studies above were observed with just 1 tbsp (7 g) of ground flaxseed per day. However, "it's best to limit your intake to around 4–5 tablespoons (28–35 grams) of flaxseed per day — so you don't get too much fiber — and enjoy as part of a healthy, balanced diet" (7), But, for everything you've always wanted to know about flaxseed, you can find out all about it on the website of the US Department of Agriculture (USDA), Agricultural Research Service, Seeds, Flaxseed, at https://fdc.nal.usda.gov/fdc-app.html#/food-details/ 169414/nutrients (accessed March 1, 2022).

The LIVESTRONG website proposes that you consume

> 3 to 4 tablespoons of flaxseed daily to benefit from the fiber and omega-3 fatty acids. If you are taking flaxseed for constipation, consume 2 tablespoons daily—toddlers should consume about 1 tablespoon per day. While there are no reports of flaxseed overdosing, you may experience excess gas and bloating if you eat large servings of the meal because of its fiber and fat content.
>
> **(8)**

*Web*MD heralds the wonderful benefits of flaxseed for the usual medical disorders but nowhere on that website are we told how much to take (9). But the Cleveland Clinic tells readers that eating 2 tbsp of ground flaxseed per day is considered a healthy daily amount (10).

What we learn from these—and other— nutrition advice websites, by inference, is that there is no systematic research leading to a Recommended Dietary Allowance (RDA) for flaxseed or flax oil, and that 1–2, but less than 5 tbsp per day is thought by many experts to be adequate.

However, the website Healthyflax.org apparently "partnering" with the Flax Council of Canada, Saskatchewan Flax Development Commission and the Manitoba Flax Growers Association tells us that

> The Institute of Medicine set the Adequate Intake of ALA at 1.6 g/day for men and 1.1 g/day for women, or 0.6–1.2% of energy intake, with a dietary omega-6 to omega-3 ratio of 5:1 to 10:1 … Eating 5 g of flaxseed oil (less than a tablespoon) or 8 g of milled flaxseed (one tablespoon) daily provides enough ALA to meeting the Adequate Intake (11).

Parenthetically, the Institute of Medicine (IOM) (of Canada) is apparently an independent branch of that nation's National Academies of Sciences, Engineering and Medicine.

Given those flaxseed or flax oil dosage guidelines for health maintenance, what are the dosage guidelines for supplementation in the case of medical disorders, where warranted and advisable? We will answer that. But first ...

6.3 CYANOGENIC GLYCOSIDES (CNGS)

Concerns have been raised about the safety of consuming flaxseed—even in normal amounts—because it contains cyanogenic glycosides (CNGs). There are only minute amounts of cyanogenic glycosides in the flaxseed and flax-containing foods we are likely to consume. CNGs are a group of plant nitrate-derived compounds that can yield cyanide following their breakdown by digestive acids and enzymes. They constitute an essential component of plant defenses against predatory microbes, fungi and viruses. There are at least 2,000 plant species that contain CNGs.

Simply put, CNGs are a combination of cyanide and sugars present in many edible plants (12) including corn, paddy rice, barley, wheat, rye, sugar cane, mango, cassava, lima beans, bamboo shoots, sorghum, flax and common fruits such as apples, and stone fruits like peaches, plums, cherries and apricots. Other sources of dietary cyanide include vitamin B12.

Although cyanide, *per se*, is a well-known poison, it is harmless when it is formed from CNGs in the minute quantities found in certain quite common foods. When CNGs are simply part of the foods consumed, or in the quantity ordinarily contained in recommended servings of flaxseeds or flaxseed oil as nutrient supplements, it is generally considered quite safe to consume it. Countless, perhaps millions of, people worldwide regularly consume flaxseeds or flaxseed oil every day ... and "live to talk about it"—in fact, to acclaim its health benefits.

The CNGs in flaxseeds are essentially the same compounds found in *amygdalin* typically extracted from apricot kernels or the synthetic form, laetrile, alleged in the 1950s to cure cancer (and now banned by the FDA). According to a report published in 2017 in the journal *Archives in Cancer Research*, when amygdalin was orally administered to people, the toxic dose was found to be 4 g per day, for 15 days (13). That dosage is vastly greater than the amount in a typical serving of flaxseed.

Estimates of the actual weight in 1 tbsp of ground flaxseed vary somewhat from source to source, but 6–7 g is the consensus; and CNGs are only a very small part of that. A report in the journal *Nutrients* tells us that no increase in plasma cyanide levels above baseline have been observed with the consumption of 15–100 g of flaxseeds—which translates to about 2–16 tbsp (14).

According to a 2019 report in the *Journal of Food Science and Technology*, 1–2 tbsp of flaxseed will produce only approximately 5–10 mg of hydrogen cyanide after ingestion. This is highly unlikely to cause toxicity because (A) a 50–60 mg dose of cyanide is required to cause acute toxicity; and (B) the human body can routinely detoxify up to 100 mg/day of cyanide (15, 16) and, by the way, cyanide is heat labile and in cooking foods, it is destroyed (17).

In a study published in the *American Journal of Physiology. Heart and Circulatory Physiology* in 2018, it was reported that people given 50 g/day flaxseeds did not show increased urinary levels of *thiocyanate*, a signature metabolite of cyanide (15). Based on these data, people would need to consume the unrealistic amount of 1 kilogram (kg) (2.2 pounds (lb)) of flaxseeds daily for cyanide toxicity to develop (18). For comparison, the average box of cereal might contain about 16 oz (1 lb) of cereal, net weight. So, to get to the 2.2 lb threshold, one would have to consume a staggering quantity of about two (2) entire cereal boxes worth of flaxseed, per day, to begin to reach a level of toxicity.

The recommendation of daily dietary supplementation of 9 g of flaxseed was reported in the *Journal of Food Science and Technology* in connection with its high content of ALA (flaxseeds hold about 23 g of ALA/100 g) (19). However, Healthline stipulates that supplementation should be kept below 5 tbsp per day (20). And The Flax Council of Canada reports that consumption of moderate amounts of flaxseed (1 to 2 tbsp) daily is not likely to pose a health problem for North Americans who have adequate intakes of protein and iodine (21).

In a study published in the *British Journal of Nutrition* in 1993, it was reported that volunteers ate muffins containing 50 g (5–6 tbsp) of milled flax daily for up to 6 weeks, without ill effects. However, it should be noted that muffins made with milled flax showed no trace of the CNGs—confirming that cooking destroyed the CNGs (22).

To sum up: The acute lethal oral dose of cyanide in humans is reported to be between 0.5 and 3.5 mg/kg body weight. The toxic threshold value for cyanide in blood is considered to be between 0.5 (ca 20 micromoles (μmol)) and 1.0 mg/liter (L) (ca 40 μmol). The lethal threshold value ranges between 2.5 (ca 100 μmol) and 3.0 mg/L (ca 120 μmol). So, 120 g of crushed/ground flaxseed can be consumed before a toxic threshold of 40 μmol/L is reached (23). A tablespoon of milled flaxseed weighs about 10 g. Thus, to approach the toxic threshold of 40 μmol/L, one would have to consume about 12 tbsp of milled flaxseed at a sitting.

Furthermore, the safety and benefits of flaxseed are so well established that it is recommended for heart health and other health reasons by numerous conventional medicine-based websites. For instance:

American Heart Association News. Know the flax (and the chia): A little seed may be what your diet needs (July 19, 2019): "Flaxseeds or chia seeds offer good sources of alpha-linolenic acid (ALA), which are unsaturated fatty acids that convert to omega-3 fatty acids typically found in fish," said Linda Van Horn, a registered dietitian and professor in the department of preventive medicine at Northwestern University in Chicago. "But they also offer a good plant-based supply of plant-based proteins, fiber, minerals and other nutrients."

Mayo Clinic (by Mayo Clinic Staff): Overview— Polyunsaturated Fat:

> Flaxseed (*Linum usitatissimum*) and flaxseed oil, which comes from flaxseed, are rich sources of the essential fatty acid alpha-linolenic acid — a heart-healthy omega-3 fatty acid. Flaxseed is high in soluble fiber and in lignans, which contain phytoestrogens. Similar to the hormone estrogen, phytoestrogens might have anti-cancer properties. Flaxseed oil doesn't have these phytoestrogens.

Health experts from many leading academic centers have made strong recommendations that people use flaxseed and flaxseed oil to reduce cholesterol and blood sugar, and to treat diseases of the heart, kidneys and digestive system. A number of these experts also recommend taking flaxseed to treat inflammatory diseases such as arthritis (24).

The American Heart Association (AHA) website: "Polyunsaturated fats can have a beneficial effect on your heart when eaten in moderation and when used to replace saturated fat and trans fat in your diet." Foods high in polyunsaturated fats include a number of plant-based oils such as:

- Soybean oil.
- Corn oil.
- Sunflower oil.
- Flaxseed oil.

Other sources include some nuts and seeds such as walnuts and sunflower seeds, tofu and soybeans. The AHA also recommends eating tofu and other forms of soybeans, canola, walnut and flaxseed and their oils. These foods contain ALA, another omega-3 FA (25). And, finally from the Cleveland Clinic.

"Flaxseed: Little Seed, Big Benefits. How and why you should be adding flax to your diet":

Flaxseed benefits. Why do dietitians love flaxseed? Let us count the ways:

… Flaxseed is a good source of high-quality plant protein, comparable to soybeans. Potassium. Potassium is a mineral that's important for cell and muscle function and helps maintain normal blood pressure. But many Americans don't get enough.

Enter flaxseed, which has more potassium than (the famously potassium-rich) bananas (26).

6.4 DISCLAIMER

In the clinical and experimental (animal model) studies cited in this book, flaxseed, flaxseed oil and their individual constituents (omega-3 ALA, L-arginine and trace amounts of CNGs), with the exception of CNGs per se, and marine oil and their constituents are commonly independent treatment variables. In many cases, they are cited as adjuvant treatment for conditions ranging from heart failure to diabetes, to chronic kidney disease and inflammatory diseases.

We will list the dosages that are recommended in these studies. But for obvious professional and ethical reasons, we cite these dosages here for information purposes only. We can make no specific recommendations of any one supplement, either a flax product or one of its constituents or a marine product or one of its constituents described in this book, without competent medical or other qualified health provider supervision.

While flaxseed and its constituents, and marine foods and products are generally considered safe as food, not everyone tolerates certain foods, and allergy, even anaphylaxis. is always a possibility. There are also other cases where generally well-tolerated foods or substances can have an unpredicted paradoxical effect. In addition, flaxseed or its constituents supplemented as adjuvant treatment for a serious medical condition cannot be undertaken without exact knowledge of its safety in that setting, interactions with prescribed medications, etc. This requires on-site medical expertise. We cannot provide that.

Let's take L-arginine as an example of the above issue: Multiple myeloma is an L-arginine *auxotrophic* cancer. The tumor feeds on L-arginine. Therefore, it might be unwise to consume foods or supplements high in the amino acid L-arginine. The NutritionData website offers a list of food and their L-arginine content from highest to lowest: https://nutritiondata.self. com/foods-000089000000000000000.html; accessed February 23, 2022. L-arginine can also trigger herpes replication (oral or genital).

6.5 CAVEAT

Flaxseeds or flaxseed oil may result in lowered blood sugar. This may be of concern for individuals with diabetes controlling their blood glucose levels with prescription meds.

Consuming flaxseed oil may lower blood pressure. This may be of concern for persons who are concurrently taking anti-hypertensive meds and/or diuretics. Flaxseeds may increase the chances of bleeding. This may be of concern for persons concurrently taking certain medications such as anticoagulants or "blood thinners" including but not limited to aspirin, Coumadin, Plavix, Eliquis and Xarelto. Flaxseed and its constituents can affect hormones. This may be of concern for pregnant or lactating women.

Some people may be allergic to flaxseed or its constituents.

There is conflicting information about whether ALA in flaxseeds and flaxseed oil causes prostate cancer to become more aggressive. However, flaxseed oil contains lignans, compounds which have been linked to slowing the growth of prostate cancers.

Also, because flaxseed or its constituents can interfere with the absorption or function of other medications, that is an additional reason why consultation with a qualified healthcare provider is essential.

6.6 (ALMOST) EVERYTHING YOU'D WANT TO KNOW ABOUT FLAXSEED

How much the ALA in flaxseed or flax oil is bioavailable depends on the kind and form of flax consumed. Flaxseed oil has greater absorbability and therefore greater bioavailability than milled seed which, in turn, has greater bioavailability than whole seed (27). Crushing and milling flaxseed considerably improves the bioavailability of the enterolignans (28), likely due to the improved accessibility of the gut bacteria to crushed and ground flaxseed, the dose of flaxseed ingested (29) and the fat composition of the diet.

For instance, concurrent consumption of omega-6 linoleic acid (LA) in the diet may reduce ALA accumulation (29) because there is competition among the enzymes involved in the digestion of LA and ALA. A ratio of LA to ALA of 4:1 or lower has been shown to be optimal (30). And, neither does age appear to influence ALA bioavailability (see below) or its conversion to docosahexaenoic acid (DHA) (31); nor does gender make a difference (28). However, eicosapentaenoic acid (EPA) and DHA, found largely in marine omegas, are more rapidly incorporated into plasma and membrane lipids, and produce more rapid effects than from flaxseed ALA. Therefore, the role of ALA in human nutrition may be more important in terms of long-term dietary intake (32).

When one consumes foods or nutrient supplements, one does so assuming that the body will absorb them and that they will become "bioavailable," meaning that the body will be able to put them to work. So, how absorbable is flaxseed, and how bioavailable are its constituents?

According to a 2008 report in the *Journal of the American College of Nutrition*, 30 g of seed, or 6 g of ALA in the oil, were baked into muffins for consumption over a 3-month test period by healthy men and women. Consumption over a 1-month period resulted in significant increases in plasma ALA levels in the flaxseed oil and the milled flaxseed-supplemented groups. The flaxseed oil group had significantly higher ALA levels than the milled flaxseed group. The participants who supplemented with whole flaxseed did not see a significant increase in plasma ALA levels.

Participants in all of the groups had some symptoms of gastrointestinal discomfort during the early stages of the study but these disappeared in both the oil and the milled seed groups.

The investigators concluded that consuming flax oil and milled flaxseed raises plasma ALA levels, whereas whole flaxseed does not. Whole seed and oil preparations can induce adverse gastrointestinal effects within 4 weeks causing some participants to withdraw from the study, but no one withdrew from the group that ingested milled flaxseed and, therefore, that may represent a good form of flaxseed to avoid side effects and still provide significant increases in ALA to the body (27).

Another question is whether the person's age affects bioavailability. The aim of a study published in 2009 in the *European Journal of Clinical Nutrition* was to determine whether there is an age difference in the response to a diet containing 6 g of ALA from ground flaxseed or 30 g of flaxseed oil over a period of 4 weeks, in participants 18 to 29 years old, or in participants 45 to 69 years old. It was found that age does not determine ALA absorption from a flaxseed-supplemented diet nor in the metabolism of ALA to EPA when consuming flaxseed oil. However, younger participants, but not the older ones, derived a beneficial decrease in circulating triglycerides from flaxseed supplementation (31).

Flaxseed is one of the richest sources of lignans and is increasingly used in food products or as a supplement. Plant lignans can be converted by intestinal bacteria into the so-called enterolignans, enterodiol and enterolactone. There is evidence that these reduce the risk of coronary heart disease and risk of death (33). For a proper evaluation of potential health effects of enterolignans, information on their bioavailability is essential. Therefore, the question is whether crushing and milling of flaxseed substantially improve the bioavailability of the enterolignans.

Therefore, a study published in 2005 in the *Journal of Nutrition* aimed to determine whether crushing and milling of flaxseed enhances the bioavailability of enterolignans in plasma. Healthy participants supplemented their diet with 0.3 g of whole, crushed or ground flaxseed/kg body weight per day for ten consecutive days, separated by a wash-out period where the participants held to a diet poor in lignans. It was found that the average bioavailability of enterolignans from ground flaxseed, 43%, was significantly greater than that from whole flaxseed 28% (28).

Table 6.1 compares ALA content in different foods.

6.6.1 Supplement Dosages in Published Clinical Trials

Only clinical trials, i.e., research involving human participants, are reported here. There are many valuable research trials, i.e., animal model trials (rats, mice, rabbits), that reveal the benefits of flax supplementation, but dosages do not translate in any useful way to human application.

Were one to suffer any chronic inflammation, even absent cardiovascular or related disease, it is unimaginable that there isn't already some serious damage to the endothelial lining of the blood vessels—body-wide. With that in mind, two major and one minor constituent of flaxseed address the problem of endothelial impairment and nitric oxide (NO) unavailability: Omega-3 and 6 FAs; L-arginine and CNGs.

First, although CNGs are NO donors—digestion results in NO formation—they likely play little if any role in the beneficial effects of flaxseed. They don't actually produce much in amounts that would be helpful here. Second, because of the current popular focus of research on the effects of antioxidant omega-3 FAs, it is in most cases not possible to extricate the role played by L-arginine from the effects attributed to omega-3s. Increased NO availability is simply embedded in the results.

But, in sum, there is strong evidence that the constituents of flaxseed, individually or altogether, promote cardiovascular health by supporting endothelium viability and/or supplying L-arginine for NO formation. So, the two main relevant ingredients in flaxseed and flaxseed oil supplementation are the omega-3 and -6 FAs and L-arginine (about 2 g of L-arginine per 100 g of flaxseed). We therefore list here examples of the published range of dosages of flaxseed or flax oil, *per se*, in selected clinical trials and there are, by the way, no published dosages for the use of CNGs in adjuvant treatment of any conventional relevant medical condition.

It is possible that one may be considering supplementation of flaxseed or flax oil because of a medical condition that perhaps could be helped by such supplementation. So that one can consult with the health services professional of choice, we supply here information about some common conditions, the treatment dosage, the title of the study, the journal in which the study was published and year of publication. This should help, in consultation with one's healthcare provider, to determine whether such supplementation is appropriate. Please note that the simplest and most direct way to access a given report is by entering the Digital Object Identifier (DOI) and if that is not available, the PubMed reference number (PMID).

TABLE 6.1
Selected Sources of Alpha-Linolenic Acid (ALA) and Content of ALA in Selected Novel Sources of Omega-3 Polyunsaturated Fatty Acids [1 tbsp oil = 13.6 g; 1 tbsp seeds or nuts = 12.35 g]

Source of ALA[a]	ALA Content, g
Pumpkin seeds (1 tbsp)	0.051
Olive oil (1 tbsp)	0.103
Walnuts, black (1 tbsp)	0.156
Soybean oil (1 tbsp)	1.231
Rapeseed oil (1 tbsp)	1.302
Walnut oil (1 tbsp)	1.414
Flaxseeds (1 tbsp)	2.350
Walnuts, English (1 tbsp)	2.574
Flaxseed oil (1 tbsp)	**7.249**
Almonds (100 g)	0.4
Peanuts (100 g)	0.003
Beans, navy, sprouted (100 g)	0.3
Broccoli, raw (100 g)	0.1
Lettuce, red leaf (100 g)	0.1
Mustard (100 g)	0.1
Purslane (100 g)	0.4
Spinach (100 g)	0.1
Seaweed, spirulina, dried (100 g)	0.8
Beans, common, dry (100 g)	0.6
Chickpeas, dry (100 g)	0.1
Soybeans, dry (100 g)	1.6
Oats, germ (100 g)	1.4
Rice, bran (100 g)	0.2
Wheat, germ (100 g)	0.7
Avocados, California, raw (100 g)	0.1
Raspberries, raw (100 g)	0.1
Strawberries, raw (100 g)	0.1
Breads and pasta (100 g)	0.1–1.6
Cereals (and granola bars) (55 g)	1.0–4.9
Eggs (50 g or 1 egg)	0.1–0.6
Processed meats (100 g)	0.5
Salad dressing (14–31 g)	2.0–4.0
Margarine spreads (10–100 g)	0.3–1.0
Nutrition bars (50 g)	0.1–2.2

[a] Adapted from Kris-Etherton, Taylor, Yu-Poth et al. 2000 (34) and Gebauer, Psota, Harris et al. 2006 (35).
Source: Adapted from Whelan and Rust. 2006 (36).

Most people may turn to flaxseed for prevention and the thing that it is most important to prevent is, of course, chronic systemic inflammation. It precedes, and likely it may even cause, everything one might wind up coming down with, such as hypertension, atherosclerosis, Type 2 diabetes and heart and kidney disease. You may recall that what chronic inflammation does, up front, is serious damage to the endothelium.

6.7 CHRONIC SYSTEMIC INFLAMMATION

For all of the disease conditions that follow, the main purpose of listing them is simply to show the approximate dosage that was used in the studies. Therefore, while we are presenting the title of the studies, we are not, in these following sections, reviewing and summarizing the results as we had done in earlier sections of this chapter. Again, we just want to pinpoint the dosage.

The Arthritis Foundation, Living with Arthritis Blog features "Anti-Inflammatory Benefits of Flaxseed": Just 2 tbsp of ground flaxseed contain more than 140% of the daily value of the inflammation-reducing omega-3 FAs, plus more lignans, a cancer-fighting plant chemical, than any other plant food on the planet …. In a study where volunteers consumed flaxseed oil for 4 weeks, the ALAs significantly decreased pro-inflammatory mediators ….

As noted previously, there are a number of ways to consume flaxseed. The Arthritis Foundation lists the following "8 Ways to Get Your Flaxseed:"

- Stir 1 tbsp of ground flaxseed into oatmeal, cereal and smoothies.
- Use ground flaxseed as a topping for salads.
- Make vinaigrette with 1 tbsp Dijon mustard, 1 tbsp vinegar and 3 tbsp flaxseed oil.
- Mix 1 tbsp ground flaxseed into tuna, chicken and egg salads.
- Add ¼ cup whole or ground flaxseed to bread recipes.
- Toss ½ lb cooked pasta with 2 tbsp flaxseed oil.
- Coat and roast vegetables in equal parts flaxseed and olive oil.
- Replace half the oil or butter in baking recipes with flaxseed oil (37).

6.8 INFLAMMATION IN METABOLIC SYNDROME (READ ENDOTHELIAL DYSFUNCTION)

Dosage: 25 milliliters (mL)/day flaxseed oil. As reported in a clinical study titled "A comparative study of the effect of flaxseed oil and sunflower oil on the Coagulation Score, selected oxidative and inflammatory parameters in metabolic syndrome patients," published in 2020 in the journal *Clinical Nutrition Research* (38).

6.8.1 Metabolic Syndrome

Dosage: Flaxseed lignan (543 mg/day^{-1} in a 4,050 mg complex). As reported in a clinical study titled "A randomized controlled trial of the effects of flaxseed lignan complex on metabolic syndrome composite score and bone mineral in older adults," published in 2009, in the journal *Applied Physiology, Nutrition and Metabolism* (39).

6.9 INFLAMMATION IN ULCERATIVE COLITIS

Dosage: Group 1—30 g/day of ground flaxseed; and Group 2—10 g/day of ground flaxseed for 12 weeks. Reported in a study titled "Effects of flaxseed and flaxseed oil supplement on serum levels of inflammatory markers, metabolic parameters and severity of disease in patients with ulcerative colitis," published in the journal *Complementary Therapies in Medicine*, in 2019 (40).

6.10 CARDIOVASCULAR RISK FACTORS

Dosage: 40 g/day of ground flaxseed-containing baked products. Reported in the *Journal of the American College of Nutrition* in 2008, in a study titled "Flaxseed and cardiovascular risk factors: Results from a double blind, randomized, controlled clinical trial" (41).

6.11 CORONARY ARTERY DISEASE

Dosage: 12 weeks consumption of flaxseed (30 g/day) vs usual care control. As reported in 2019 in a clinical trial in the *European Journal of Clinical Nutrition* titled "Effect of flaxseed consumption on flow-mediated dilation and inflammatory biomarkers in patients with coronary artery disease: A randomized controlled trial" (Read Endothelial Dysfunction) (42).

6.12 ABNORMAL SERUM LIPIDS

Dosage: 30 g (3 tbsp equiv.) [per day] of roasted flaxseed powder for 3 months. As reported in 2014 in a clinical study titled "Evaluation of flaxseed formulation as a potential therapeutic agent in mitigation of dyslipidemia," published in 2014 in the *Biomedical Journal* (43).

6.13 CARDIOVASCULAR RISK FACTORS

Dosage: At least 500 mg of the lignan SDG/day for approximately 8 weeks. Reported in a 2010 clinical study titled "Health effects with consumption of the flax lignan secoisolariciresinol diglucoside," in the *British Journal of Nutrition* (44).

6.14 TYPE 2 DIABETES

Dosage: 10 g of flaxseed per day for 1 month. As reported in a clinical study titled "An open-label study on the effect of flaxseed powder (*Linum usitatissimum*) supplementation in the management of diabetes mellitus" published in 2011 in the *Journal of Dietary Supplements* (45).

6.14.1 TYPE 2 DIABETES WITH MILD HYPERCHOLESTEROLEMIA

Dosage: Flaxseed-derived lignan capsules (360 mg lignan per day) for 12 weeks separated by an 8-week wash-out period. Reported in 2007 in a clinical study titled "Effects of a flaxseed-derived lignan supplement in type 2 diabetic patients: A randomized, double-blind, cross-over trial," published in the journal *PLoS One* (46).

6.15 LUPUS NEPHRITIS

Dosage: 15, 30 and 45 g of flaxseed/day sequentially at 4-week intervals. Reported in 1995 in the journal *Kidney International* in a report titled "Flaxseed: A potential treatment for lupus nephritis" (47).

6.16 OBESITY AND INSULIN RESISTANCE

Dosage: 40 g of ground flaxseed per day. Reported in 2011 in a study published in the *Nutrition Journal* titled "Flaxseed supplementation improved insulin resistance in obese glucose intolerant people: A randomized crossover design" (48).

6.17 SYSTEMIC INFLAMMATION IN MORBID OBESITY

Dosage: Flaxseed flour (Farinha de Linhaca Dourada LinoLive, Cisbra, Brazil) in the amount of 30 g/day. Reported in the journal *Obesity Surgery* in 2007, in a study titled "Systemic inflammation in morbidly obese subjects: Response to oral supplementation with alpha-linolenic acid" (49).

6.18 PROSTATE CANCER

Dosage: 30 g/day flaxseed-supplemented diet. Reported in 2008 in a study titled "Flaxseed supplementation (not dietary fat restriction) reduces prostate cancer proliferation rates in men presurgery," in the journal *Cancer Epidemiology, Biomarkers and Prevention* (50).

6.19 RHEUMATOID ARTHRITIS

Dosage: A daily dose of 3 g of EPA and DHA per day for 12 weeks or more. As reported in 2000 in a clinical study titled "n−3 fatty acid supplements in rheumatoid arthritis" (51).

6.20 OSTEOARTHRITIS—FLAXSEED POULTICE COMPRESS

Dosage: The poultice was applied once a day for 7 days in a row. Reported in 2019 in a publication in the journal *Clinical Rheumatology*, titled "Effect of flaxseed poultice compress application on pain and hand functions of patients with hand osteoarthritis" (52).

6.21 CHRONIC KIDNEY DISEASE

There are many recent publications reporting the benefits of omega FAs derived from marine sources in ameliorating chronic kidney disease. They can be found in a previous chapter. But there are no recent studies of the benefits of flaxseed or flax oil in human kidney disease. Medical journal publications report treatment in animal models (mice, rats, rabbits).

6.22 CHRONIC KIDNEY DISEASE: INFLAMMATION AND OXIDATIVE STRESS IN HEMODIALYSIS

Dosage: The patients in the flaxseed oil group received 6 g/day flaxseed oil for 8 weeks. As reported in 2016 in the journal *International Urology and Nephrology*, in a clinical study titled "Effect of flaxseed oil on serum systemic and vascular inflammation markers and oxidative stress in hemodialysis patients: A randomized controlled trial" (53).

6.23 POLYCYSTIC OVARY SYNDROME

Dosage: 30 g/day. Reported in the *Nutrition Journal* in 2020, in a clinical study titled "The effects of flaxseed supplementation on metabolic status in women with polycystic ovary syndrome: A randomized open-labeled controlled clinical trial" (54).

6.23.1 Hormonal Levels in Polycystic Ovarian Syndrome

Dosage: 30 g/day. Reported in 2007 in the journal *Current Topics in Nutraceutical Research* in a study titled "The effect of flaxseed supplementation on hormonal levels associated with polycystic ovarian syndrome: A case study" (55).

The brief listings above are intended to illustrate the range of dosages that clinical investigators consider safe as a medical treatment in a sample of differing applications. Bear in mind that clinical application dosages can differ significantly from supplements intended to benefit health absent a serious medical disorder.

REFERENCES

1. Herchi W, Arráez-Román D, Trabelsi H, Bouali I, Boukhchina B, Kallel H, Segura-Carretero A, and A Fernández-Gutierrez. 2014. Phenolic compounds in flaxseed: a review of their properties and analytical methods. An overview of the last decade. *Journal of Oleo Science*, 63(1): 7–14. DOI: 10.5650/jos.ess13135.
2. Prasad K, and A Jadhav. 2016. Prevention and treatment of atherosclerosis with flaxseed-derived compound secoisolariciresinol diglucoside. *Current Pharmaceutical Design*, 22(2): 214–220. DOI: 10.2174/1381612822666151112151130.
3. Simopoulos AP. 2000. Human requirement for N-3 polyunsaturated fatty acids. *Poultry Science*, Jul; 79(7): 961–970. DOI: 10.1093/ps/79.7.961.
4. Francois CA, Connor SL, Bolewicz LC, and WE Connor. 2003. Supplementing lactating women with flaxseed oil does not increase docosahexaenoic acid in their milk. *American Journal of Clinical Nutrition, Jan*; 77(1): 226–233. DOI: 10.1093/ajcn/77.1.226.

5. https://www.mayoclinichealthsystem.org/hometown-health/speaking-of-health/flaxseed-is-nutritionally-powerful#:~:text=While%20there%20are%20no%20specific,2%20grams%20of%20dietary%20fiber; accessed 3/1/22.
6. https://www.medicinenet.com/how_much_flaxseed_should_you_eat_a_day/ article.htm; accesed 3/1/22.
7. https://www.healthline.com/nutrition/benefits-of-flaxseeds#TOC_TITLE_HDR_2; accessed 3/1/22.
8. https://www.livestrong.com/article/456688-the-dosage-of-ground-flaxseed/; accessed 3/1/22.
9. https://www.webmd.com/diet/features/benefits-of-flaxseed; accessed 3/1/22.
10. https://my.clevelandclinic.org/health/articles/17651-plant-sources-of-omega-3s#:~:text=Eating%202%20Tablespoons%20of%20ground,considered%20a%20healthy%20daily%20amount.&text=Because%20flaxseed%20is%20high%20in,become%20rancid%20or%20spoil%20quickly; accessed 3/1/22.
11. https://www.healthyflax.org/contact/index.php; accessed 3/1/22.
12. Bolarinwa IF, Oke MO, Olaniyan SA, and AS Ajala. 2016. *A review of cyanogenic glycosides in edible plants.* IntechOpen—Toxicology, October 26. DOI: 10.5772/ 64886.
13. Qadir M, and K Fatima. 2017. Review on pharmacological activity of amygdalin. *Archives in Cancer Research*, 5(4): 160. DOI: 10.21767/2254-6081.100160.
14. Cressey P, and J Reeve. 2019. Metabolism of cyanogenic glycosides: A review. *Food and Chemical Toxicology*, Mar; 125: 225–232. DOI: 10.1016/j.fct.2019. 01.002.
15. Parikh M, Netticadan T, and GB Pierce. 2018. Flaxseed: Its bioactive components and their cardiovascular benefits. *American Journal of Physiology. Heart and Circulation Physiology*, Feb; 314(2): H146–H159. DOI: 10.1152/ajpheart.00 400.2017.
16. Touré A, and X Xueming. 2019. Flaxseed lignans: Source, biosynthesis, metabolism, antioxidant activity, bio-active components, and health benefits. *Comprehensive Reviews in Food Science and Food Safety*, May; 9: 261–269. DOI: 10.1111/j.1541-4337.2009.00105.x.
17. Kajla P, Sharma and DR Sood. 2015. Flaxseed—A potential functional food source. *Journal of Food Science and Technology*, Apr; 52(4): 1857–1871. DOI: 10.1007/s13197-014-1293-y.
18. Parikh M, Maddaford TG, Austria A, Aliani M, Netticadan T, and GN Pierce1. 2019. Dietary flaxseed as a strategy for improving human health. *Nutrients, May*; 11(5): 1171. DOI: 10.3390/nu11051171.
19. Goyal A, Sharma V, Upadhyay N, Gill S, and M Sihag. 2014. Flax and flaxseed oil: An ancient medicine and modern functional food. *Journal of Food Science and Technology*, Sep; 51(9): 1633–1653. DOI: 10.1007/s13197-013-1247-9.
20. https://www.healthline.com/nutrition/benefits-of-flaxseeds; accessed 1/7/21.
21. Morris DH, 2007. *F LAX – A health and nutrition primer.* Fourth ed. Chapter 8: Safety of Flax; https://flaxcouncil.ca/wp-content/uploads/2015/03/FlxPrmr_4ed_ Chpt8.pdf.
22. Cunnane SC, Ganguli S, Menard C, Liede AC, Hamadeh MJ, Chen ZY, Wolever TM, and DJ Jenkins. 1993. High α-linolenic acid flaxseed (*Linum usitatissimum*): Some nutritional properties in humans. *British Journal of Nutrition*, 69: 443–453. DOI: 10.1079/bjn19930046.
23. Schrenk D, Bignami M, Bodin L, Kevin Chipman JK, del Mazo J, Grasl-Kraupp B, Hogstrand C, Hoogenboom L(R), Leblanc J-C, Nebbia CS, Nielsen E, Ntzani E, Petersen A, Sand S, Vleminckx C, Wallace H, Benford D, Brimer L, Mancini FR, Metzler M, Viviani B, Altieri A, Arcella D, Steinkellner H, and T Schwerdtle. 2019. Evaluation of the health risks related to the presence of cyanogenic glycosides in foods other than raw apricot kernels: EFSA Panel on Contaminants in the Food Chain (CONTAM), *European Food Safety Authority*, 17(4): 5662. DOI: 10.2903/j.efsa. 2019.5662.

24. https://www.mayoclinic.org/drugs-supplements-flaxseed-and-flaxseed-oil/art-20366457; accessed 5/12/21.
25. https://www.heart.org/en/healthy-living/healthy-eating/eat-smart/fats/polyunsaturated-fats; accessed 11/15/21.
26. https://health.clevelandclinic.org/flaxseed-little-seed-big-benefits/; accessed 11/15/21.
27. Austria JA, Richard MN, Chahine MN, Edel AL, Malcolmson LJ, Dupasquier CMC, and GN Pierce. 2008. Bioavailability of alpha-linolenic acid in subjects after ingestion of three different forms of flaxseed. *Journal of the American College of Nutrition*, Apr; 27(2): 214–221. DOI: 10.1080/07315724.2008.10719693.
28. Kuijsten A, Art ICW, van't Veer P, and PCH Hollman. 2005. The relative bioavailability of enterolignans in humans is enhanced by milling and crushing of flaxseed. *Journal of Nutrition*, Dec; 135(12): 2812–2816. DOI: 10.1093/jn/135.12. 2812.
29. Arterburn LM, Hall EB, and H Oken. 2006. Distribution, interconversion, and dose response of n-3 fatty acids in humans. *American Journal of Clinical Nutrition*, Jun; 83(6 Suppl) Suppl: 1467S–1476S. DOI: 10.1093/ajcn/83.6.1467S.
30. Ghafoorunissa IMM. 1992. n-3 fatty acids in Indian diets—Comparison of the effects of precursor (alpha-linolenic acid) vs product (long chain n-3 poly unsaturated fatty acids). *Nutrition Research*, Apr–May; 12(4–5): 569–582. DOI: 10.1016 / S0271-5317(05)80027-2.
31. Patenaude A, Rodriguez-Leyva D, Edel AL, Dibrov E, Dupasquier CMC, Austria JA, Richard MN, Chahine MN, Malcolmson LJ, and GN Pierce. 2009. Bioavailability of alpha-linolenic acid from flaxseed diets as a function of the age of the subject. *European Journal of Clinical Nutrition*, Sep; 63(9): 1123–1129. DOI: 10.1038/ ejcn.2009.41.
32. Rodriguez-Leyva D, Bassett CMC, McCullough R, and GN Pierce. 2010. The cardiovascular effects of flaxseed and its omega-3 fatty acid, alpha-linolenic acid. *Canadian Journal of Cardiology*, Nov; 26(9): 489–496. DOI: 10.1016/s0828-282x(10)70455-4.
33. Peterson J, Dwyer J, Adlercreutz H, Scalbert A, Jacques P, and ML McCulloug. 2010. Dietary lignans: Physiology and potential for cardiovascular disease risk reduction. *Nutrition Reviews*, Oct; 68(10): 571–603. DOI: 10.1111/j.1753-4887.2010.00319.x.
34. Kris-Etherton PM, Taylor DS, Yu-Poth S, Huth P, Moriarty K, Fishell V, Hargrove RL, Zhao G, and TD Etherton. 2000. Polyunsaturated fatty acids in the food chain in the United States. *American Journal of Clinical Nutrition, Jan*; 71(1 Suppl) Suppl: 179S–1788S. DOI: 10.1093/ajcn/71.1.179S.
35. Gebauer SK, Psota TL, Harris WS, and PM Kris-Etherton. 2006. n-3 fatty acid dietary recommendations and food sources to achieve essentiality and cardiovascular benefits. *American Journal of Clinical Nutrition, Jun*; 83(6 Suppl) Suppl: 1526S–1535S. DOI: 10.1093/ajcn/83.6.1526S.
36. Whelan J, and C Rust. 2006. Innovative dietary sources of n-3 fatty acids. *Annual Review of Nutrition*, 26: 75–103. DOI: 10.1146/annurev.nutr.25.050304.092605.
37. http://blog.arthritis.org/living-with-arthritis/health-benefits-flaxseed-anti-inflammatory/; accessed 2/27/22.
38. Akrami A, Makiabadi E, Askarpour M, Zamani K, Hadi A, Mokari-Yamchi A, Babajafari S, Faghih S, and A Hojhabrimanesh. 2020. A comparative study of the effect of flaxseed oil and sunflower oil on the Coagulation Score, selected oxidative and inflammatory parameters in metabolic syndrome patients. *Clinical Nutrition Research, Jan*; 9(1): 63–72. DOI: 10.7762/cnr.2020.9.1.63.
39. Cornish SM, Chilibeck PD, Paus-Jennsen L, Biem HJ, Khozani T, Senanayake V, Vatanparast H, Little JP, Whiting SJ, and P Pahwa. 2009. A randomized controlled trial of the effects of flaxseed lignan complex on metabolic syndrome Composite Score and bone mineral in older adults. *Applied Physiology, Nutrition and Metabolism*, Apr; 34(2): 89–98. DOI: 10.1139/H08-142.

40. Morshedzadeh N, Shahrokh S, Aghdaei HA, Pourhoseingholi MA, Chaleshi V, Hekmatdoost A, Karimi S, Zali MR, and P Mirmiran. 2019. Effects of flaxseed and flaxseed oil supplement on serum levels of inflammatory markers, metabolic parameters and severity of disease in patients with ulcerative colitis. *Complementary Therapies in Medicine*, Oct; 46: 36–43. DOI: 10.1016/j.ctim.2019.07.012.
41. Bloedon LT, Balikai S, Chittams J, Cunnane SC, Berlin JA, Rader DJ, and PO Szapary. 2008. Flaxseed and cardiovascular risk factors: results from a double blind, randomized, controlled clinical trial. *Journal of the American College of Nutrition*, Feb; 27(1): 65–74. DOI: 10.1080/07315724.2008.10719676.
42. Khandouzi N, Zahedmehr A, Mohammadzadeh A, Sanati HR, and J Nasrollahzadeh. 2019. Effect of flaxseed consumption on flow-mediated dilation and inflammatory biomarkers in patients with coronary artery disease: A randomized controlled trial. *European Journal of Clinical Nutrition*, Feb; 73(2): 258–265. DOI: 10.1038/s41430-018-0268-x.
43. Saxena S, and C Katare. 2014. Evaluation of flaxseed formulation as a potential therapeutic agent in mitigation of dyslipidemia. *Biomedical Journal*, Nov–Dec; 37(6): 386–90. DOI: 10.4103/2319-4170.126447.
44. Adolphe JL, Whiting SJ, Juurlink BHJ, Thorpe LU, and J Alcorn. 2010. Health effects with consumption of the flax lignan secoisolariciresinol diglucoside. *British Journal of Nutrition*, Apr; 103(7):929–938. DOI: 10.1017/S0007114509992753.
45. Mani UV, Mani I, Biswas M, and SN Kumar. 2011. An open-label study on the effect of flax seed powder (*Linum usitatissimum*) supplementation in the management of diabetes mellitus. *Journal of Dietary Supplements*, Sep; 8(3): 257–265. DOI: 10.31 09/19390211.2011.593615.
46. Pan A, Sun J, Chen Y, Ye X, Li H, Yu Z, Wang Y, Gu W, Zhang X, Chen X, Demark-Wahnefried W, Liu Y, and X Lin. 2007. Effects of a flaxseed-derived lignan supplement in type 2 diabetic patients: A randomized, double-blind, cross-over trial. *PLoS One*, Nov 7; 2(11): e1148. DOI: 10.1371/journal.pone.0001148.
47. Clark WF, Parbtani A, Huff MW, Spanner E, De Saus H, Chin-Yee I, Philbrick J, and BJ Holub. 1995. Flaxseed: A potential treatment for lupus nephritis. *Kidney International*, Aug; 48(2): 475–480. DOI: 10.1038/ki.1995.316.
48. Rhee Y, and A Brunt. 2011. Flaxseed supplementation improved insulin resistance in obese glucose intolerant people: A randomized crossover design. *Nutrition Journal*, 10: 44. DOI: 10.1186/1475-2891-10-44.
49. Faintuch J, Horie LM, Barbeiro HV, Barbeiro DF, Soriano FG, Ishida RK, and I Cecconello. 2007, Systemic inflammation in morbidly obese subjects: Response to oral supplementation with alpha-linolenic acid. *Obesity Surgery*, Mar; 17(3): 341–347. DOI: 10.1007/s11695-007-9062-x.
50. Demark-Wahnefried W, Polascik TJ, George SL, Switzer BR, Madden JF, Ruffin MT4th, Snyder DC, Owzar K, Hars V, Albala DM, Walther PJ, Robertson CN, Moul JW, Dunn BK, Brenner D, Minasian L, Stella P, RT Vollmer. 2008. Flaxseed supplementation (not dietary fat restriction) reduces prostate cancer proliferation rates in men presurgery. *Cancer Epidemiology, Biomarkers and Prevention*, Dec; 17(12): 3577–3587. DOI: 10.1158/1055-9965.EPI-08-0008.
51. Kremer JM. 2000. n−3 Fatty acid supplements in rheumatoid arthritis. *American Journal of Clinical Nutrition*, Jan; 71(1) Supplement: 349s–351s. DOI: 10.1093/ajcn/71.1.349s
52. Savaş BB, Alparslan GB, and C Korkmaz. 2019. Effect of flaxseed poultice compress application on pain and hand functions of patients with hand osteoarthritis. *Clinical Rheumatology*, Jul; 38(7): 1961–1969. DOI: 10.1007/s10067-019-04484-7.
53. Mirfatahi M, Tabibi H, Nasrollahi A, Hedayati M, and M Taghizadeh. 2016 Effect of flaxseed oil on serum systemic and vascular inflammation markers and oxidative stress in hemodialysis patients: A randomized controlled trial. *International Urology and Nephrology*, Aug; 48(8): 1335–1341. DOI: 10.1007/s11255-016-1300-5.

54. Haidari F, Banaei-Jahromi N, Zakerkish M, and K Ahmadi . 2020. The effects of flaxseed supplementation on metabolic status in women with polycystic ovary syndrome: A randomized open-labeled controlled clinical trial. *Nutrition Journal*, 19(8): 1–11. DOI: 10.11 86/s12937-020-0524-5.
55. Nowak DA, Snyder DC, Brown AJ, and W Demark-Wahnefried. 2007. The effect of flaxseed supplementation on hormonal levels associated with polycystic ovarian syndrome: A case study. *Current Topics in Nutraceutical Research*, 5(4): 177–181. PMCID: PMC2752973.

7 Flax Is Good for You—At-Home Supplementation

> Wherever flaxseed becomes a regular food item among the peoples, there will be better health.
>
> —Mohandas Gandhi

7.1 BUT, WHAT'S GOOD FOR THE GOOSE …

… may, or it may not, be good for the gander. This chapter is about supplementing flaxseed and flax oil for their reported health benefits. But we must say at the outset that while flaxseed products—which we will describe—are generally considered safe and beneficial, we cannot guarantee that they are safe or beneficial specifically for everyone. For that reason, it is solely for informational purposes that we describe the following foods and products and their use, and those descriptions are not to be construed as specific dietary recommendations for anyone in particular. To supplement or not to supplement is up to each person to decide.

Furthermore, we strongly recommend that before anyone initiates *any* supplementation, that they consult with the healthcare provider familiar with their medical history and prescription medication regimen to determine whether flaxseed products would be safe and beneficial. That said, there are numerous published daily dosages cited in connection with clinical applications throughout the book, and there are also recommendations for supplementation for better health. So, we will just reiterate a few here.

7.2 PUBLISHED SUPPLEMENTATION RECOMMENDATIONS

1. According to the National Institutes of Health (NIH), Office of Dietary Supplements, Omega-3 Fatty Acids, Fact Sheet for Consumers: How much omega-3s do I need? The report states that experts have not established recommended amounts for omega-3 fatty acids (FAs), except for alpha-linolenic acid (ALA). Average daily recommended amounts for ALA are listed in Table 7.1 in grams (g). The amount one needs depends on age and gender.

2. healthyflax.org. Ask a Flax Expert. Flax and Your Health:

   Q. What is the recommended amount of omega-3 FAs?
   A: The Institute of Medicine (presumably of Canada) set the Adequate Intake (AI) of ALA at 1.6 g/day for men and 1.1 g/day for women, or 0.6–1.2%

of energy intake, with a dietary omega-6 to omega-3 ratio of 5:1–10:1. However, the consumption of this essential FA is very inadequate in North America, with approximately 41% of adults not meeting the AI for ALA.

However, no recommended intake level has been set by the Institute of Medicine for the omega-3 FAs eicosapentaenoic acid (EPA) or docosahexaenoic acid (DHA). The reason for this is that ALA is the only true "essential" omega-3 FA in our diet. An essential nutrient (like ALA) is one that must be obtained from foods because our body cannot make it. Because EPA and DHA can be made from ALA, they are not considered "essential" nutrients in the strictest sense. Eating 5 g of flaxseed oil (less than a tablespoon [tbsp]) or 8 g of milled flaxseed (1 tbsp) per day provides enough ALA to meet the AI (1).

TABLE 7.1
Recommended Amount of ALA by Age Ranges

Life Stage	Recommended Daily Amount of ALA
Birth to 12 months[a]	0.5 g
Children 1–3 years	0.7 g
Children 4–8 years	0.9 g
Boys 9–13 years	1.2 g
Girls 9–13 years	1.0 g
Teen boys 14–18 years	1.6 g
Teen girls 14–18 years	1.1 g
Men	1.6 g
Women	1.1 g
Pregnant teens and women	1.4 g
Breastfeeding teens and women	1.3 g

Source: https://ods.od.nih.gov/factsheets/Omega3FattyAcids-Consumer/; accessed March 2, 2022. No permission required.
[a] As total omega-3s. All other values are for ALA alone.

3. Wergin A. Diabetes Education, Nutrition Mayo Clinic Health Systems, March 31, 2015. Flaxseed is nutritionally powerful: While there are no specific recommendations for flaxseed intake, 1–2 tbsp a day is considered a healthy amount. The report states that 1 tbsp of ground flaxseed contains 37 calories, 2 g of polyunsaturated fat (includes the omega-3 FAs), 0.5 g of monounsaturated fat and 2 g of dietary fiber (2).

4. How Much Flax Seed Oil Should I Use Per Day? Boyers L. March 11, 2020; Reviewed by S. Tremblay, MSc. Livestrong.com:

> Many studies on ALA, the main beneficial compound in flaxseed oil, use 600 milligrams per day. However, the current recommendation for daily ALA intake is 1,100 milligrams for women and 1,600 milligrams for men. Since 1 tablespoon of flaxseed

oil provides 730 to 1,095 usable grams of ALA, that's about all you need each day, as long as you're eating other omega-3-rich foods too (3).

5. Harvard Health Publishing, Harvard Medical School. *Heart Health—Why Not Flaxseed Oil?*

> The health benefits of fish oil are believed to derive principally from two omega-3 fats, eicosapentaenoic acid (EPA) and docosahexaenoic acid (DHA). Flaxseed oil contains a third, plant-based omega-3, alpha-linolenic acid (ALA). Other foods (especially walnuts) and oils (canola and soybean, for example) contain ALA. But at about 7 g per tablespoon, flaxseed oil is by far the richest source (4).

7.3 SUPPLEMENTATION VS ADJUNCT TREATMENT

There is a difference between supplementation and adjunct treatment. It is assumed that the individual who wants to supplement is just looking to harvest the health benefits of a given supplement, whereas in adjunct treatment (often referred to as "complementary" treatment) there is a medical prescription treatment plan in place. As noted above, supplements may interact with prescription meds, possibly with adverse consequences. Adjunct therapies are used alongside the primary treatment method to make it work better. Flax has been used as adjunct therapy in a number of serious medical conditions.

For instance, the authors of a review of clinical and research studies, titled "The effect of flaxseed in breast cancer: a literature review," published in 2018 in the journal *Frontiers in Nutrition*, report that one of the main components of flaxseed is the lignans, of which 95% are made of the predominant secoisolariciresinol diglucoside (SDG). SDG is converted into enterolactone and enterodiol, both with antiestrogen activity and structurally similar to estrogen so they can bind to cell receptors, decreasing cell growth. Some studies have shown that the intake of omega-3 FAs is related to the reduction of breast cancer risk. In animal studies, ALA has been shown to suppress growth, size and proliferation of cancer cells and also to promote the death of breast cancer cells (5).

The term "supplementation" commonly presupposes the existence of a deficit, and that deficit may or may not be evident. Supplementing vitamins, for instance, typically presupposes that the diet is lacking in them or, at least, inadequate in supplying them. So, is there an omega FAs deficit? If there isn't, supplementation may have no value. The website of the Mount Sinai Hospital—the Mount Sinai blog—acknowledges omega-3 FA deficiency: "Symptoms of omega-3 fatty acid deficiency include fatigue, poor memory, dry skin, heart problems, mood swings or depression, and poor circulation" (6).

Perhaps the terms "insufficiency" or "suboptimal" might be a better description than "deficiency" but regardless, how wide is this deficiency? In 2019, the journal *Nutrients* published a report titled "Omega-3 fatty acid intake by age, gender, and pregnancy status in the United States: National Health and Nutrition Examination Survey 2003–2014." According to the investigators, the aim of their review was to provide an updated assessment of fish and omega-3 FA intake (i.e., EPA, DHA and combined EPA + DHA) in the United States using the 2003–2014 National Health and Nutrition Examination Survey (NHANES) data.

During this period, it was found that toddlers, children and adolescents aged 1 to 19 had significantly lower omega-3 FA intake compared to adults and seniors, which remained significant after adjusting for caloric intake. Women had significantly lower omega-3 FA intake than men, and adult and senior women had significantly lower intakes compared to men in the same age categories after adjustment for energy intake. The investigators concluded that subgroups of the population have omega-3 FA intakes well below recommended levels (7).

It may be concluded from published studies that while not every source agrees on the exact criteria for what constitutes recommended omega-3 FA intake, there seems to be a general consensus that most of us just aren't getting enough in our daily diet. The case has also been made for a two-way approach to answer that question: First, an unfavorable ratio of omega-6 to omega-3 FAs usually focuses on inadequate omega-3s rather than on excess omega-6s. There are exceptions.

For instance, a review of clinical studies published in the *Journal of Nutrition and Metabolism*, in 2012, concludes that omega-6 FAs (e.g., arachidonic acid (AA)) and omega-3 FA (e.g., EPA), are precursors to "eicosanoids" which play an important role in inflammation. In general, eicosanoids derived from omega-6 FAs are pro-inflammatory, while eicosanoids derived from omega-3 FAs are anti-inflammatory.

The authors further hold that dietary changes over the past few decades show striking increases in the omega-6 to omega-3 ratio (~15:1). This change coincides with an increase in chronic inflammatory diseases including cardiovascular disease, obesity, inflammatory bowel disease (IBD), rheumatoid arthritis and Alzheimer's disease (AD) (8). The authors further state that by increasing the omega-3 to omega-6 FA ratio in our Western diet, reductions may be achieved in the incidence of these chronic inflammatory diseases. Given that the ratio is usually shown as omega-6:omega-3, and since there is a need to increase the omega-3s, therefore ideally the ratio when expressed in that sequence should be a *lower* number.

In theory, there are two ways to achieve this: lower 6 or raise 3. Most authorities propose raising 3s because, bottom line, it is not so much the ratio that counts but how many omega-3s are consumed. As noted previously, studies on the relationship between cardiovascular risks and diseases and the Omega-3 Index likewise point to widespread omega-3 FA deficits.

The authors of an extensive review of clinical and research studies titled "Dietary flaxseed as a strategy for improving human health," published in 2019 in the journal *Nature*, reported (as we have been saying throughout) that flaxseed is a rich source of the omega-3 FA ALA, the lignan secoisolariciresinol diglucoside and fiber. These compounds provide bioactivity of value to the health of animals and humans, through their anti-inflammatory action, anti-oxidative capacity and lipid-lowering properties (9).

So, the case for supplementation has been pretty well made with some guidelines, including don't tweak the ratio by simply lowering 6s but raise 3s. We *can* lower 6s by taking certain oils and nuts out of our diet, but these are good for us too, and taking them out is not recommended because omega-6s are also necessary for cardiovascular health. In fact, The National Institutes of Health (NIH) lists the AI for linoleic acid (LA), one of the main omega-6 FAs, as follows:

- Females aged 19–50: 12 g per day.
- Females aged 51 and older: 11 g per day.
- Males aged 19–50: 17 g per day.
- Males aged 51 and older: 14 g per day (10).

Some of the foods that have higher amounts of omega-6 FAs include:

- Walnuts: 10.8 g per 1-ounce (oz) serving.
- Grapeseed oil: 9.5 g per tbsp.
- Pine nuts: 9.3 g per 28-g serving.
- Sunflower seeds: 9.3 g per 1-oz serving.
- Sunflower oil: 8.9 g per tbsp.
- Corn oil: 7.3 g per tbsp.
- Cottonseed oil: 7.0 g per tbsp.
- Soybean oil: 6.9 g per tbsp.
- Mayonnaise: 5.4 g per tbsp.
- Almonds: 3.7 g per 1-oz serving.
- Tofu: 3.0 g per half cup.
- Vegetable shortening: 3.4 g per tbsp (11).

There's little reason to discard these foods from our diet, just make sure that we have plenty of omega-3s.

7.4 TRACKING OMEGA-3 FATTY ACID INTAKE: THE OMEGA-3 INDEX

It is possible to estimate the omega-6:omega-3 FA ratio of the foods we consume but it is neither practical nor for that matter is it necessary to do that. As we indicated in a previous chapter, it is much more to our advantage to determine the adequacy of our omega-3s intake by letting the cell membranes of our red blood cells reflect back to us how we are doing in that domain. That is the Omega-3 Index.

When consuming foods, some of their constituents—omega-3 FAs in this case—accumulate in cellular membranes in the body, and the content of these FAs in some of these cell membranes is generally indicative of our average daily intake (12). The Omega-3 Index test is simply a measure of the amount of the omega-3 FAs EPA and DHA in the membranes of red blood cell sampled from a drop of blood. The Omega-3 Index test yields a percentage of omega-3 out of all omega FAs, which is simply a measure of the amount of EPA and DHA in blood. The test procedures are simple:

- Collect Sample: A simple finger prick test will draw a drop of blood.
- Mail Sample: The drop is mailed to the commercial lab where omega-3 status will be assessed.

- Get Results: Results will be sent to the email address provided within 1–2 weeks.

A number of vendors offer that test. Here is a partial list:

- OmegaQuant: https://omegaquant.com/
  5009 W. 12th Street, Suite 8 Sioux Falls, SD 57106
  Phone: 1-605-271-6917
  Toll-free: 1-800-949-0632
  info @omegaquant.com
- Alkaline for Life
- Alkamind
- Better Bones Better Body
- Blue Sky Vitamins
- Carlson Labs
- Dr Guberman
- Fruugo
- Next Level Holistic Nutrition
- Nutikom
- Parasol Nutrition
- SunVital Health
- Swanson Health Products

Studies show 8% is the optimal level of omega-3. One can view a sample Omega-3 Index Basic Report at the following site: https://omegaquant.com/wp-content/uploads/2020/12/ OmegaQuant_O3basic_v15Dec2020.pdf; accessed March 13, 2022.

7.5 ORGANIC VS NON-ORGANIC FLAXSEEDS?

The choice of organic versus non-organic foods and food products is commonly a cost/benefits decision. Consumer reports tell us that organic foods tend to be somewhat more costly. They recently conducted a unique price study, comparing the cost of a market basket of organic goods such as fruits and vegetables, meat and chicken, milk and other edibles, to their non-organic counterparts, at eight different national, regional and online grocers—more than 100 product pairings in all. On average, organic foods were 47% more expensive, but the price range was wide and depending on where they shopped, they found organic foods at the same price or even less than their conventional counterparts. It seems that much depends on *where* you shop (13).

Concerning flaxseed, according to the Flax Council of Canada, all flax that is "clean and that comes from a reputable supplier" is considered to be safe for consumption. However, the average consumer has little or no way of knowing which suppliers are "reputable," all the more so if they are purchasing from a large online retailer. And given the fact that some growers might use abundant amounts of pesticides, fungicides and the like in their agricultural processes, it might be safer to purchase organic products if at all possible.

7.6 GOLDEN FLAXSEED VS BROWN FLAXSEED

The difference between golden and brown flaxseed is minimal and centers on their macronutrient and antioxidant contents. Golden flaxseed is made up of about

- 37.5% fat
- 23% protein
- 30% carbohydrate

while brown flaxseed is made up of

- 38% fat
- 24.5% protein
- 28% carbohydrate

The main difference between golden and brown flaxseed is the type of fat in each. Golden flaxseeds have more polyunsaturated FAs and less monounsaturated FAs compared to brown flaxseeds. Although small in quantity, the golden variety also has more of the two essential fats, i.e., ALA and LA present in different amounts in golden and brown flaxseed. There is more ALA in golden flaxseed than LA.

Most people who follow a Western diet typically consume too much of the omega-6 FAs like LA, and not enough omega-3 FAs like ALA. For that reason, golden flaxseed is a better choice in supplementing diet with healthy fats. However, brown flaxseed has a substantially higher concentration of antioxidants. In fact, compared to other similar seeds, like chia seeds and perilla seeds, golden flaxseeds are always the lowest in antioxidants (14). Perilla, by the way, is a kind of mint.

7.7 WHOLE FLAXSEED VS GROUND FLAXSEED OR FLAX MEAL

According to Healthline, consuming whole or ground flaxseed delivers all three major classes of macronutrients: carbohydrates, protein and fat. When comparing golden flaxseed with brown flaxseed, the exact amount of protein, fat and carbohydrates will depend on the type chosen. Most adults are likely to consume about 1 oz (28 g) of whole or ground flaxseeds per serving and, according to the US Department of Agriculture (USDA). That is about 4–5 tbsp. This amount of flaxseed contains:

- 152 calories.
- 12 g of fat.
- 8.2 g of carbohydrate, 7.8 g of which come from dietary fiber.
- 5.2 g of protein.
- 6% of the daily value (DV) for calcium.
- 9% of the DV for iron.

- 5% of the DV for potassium.
- 27% of the DV for magnesium.
- 15% of the DV for phosphorus.
- 11% of the DV for zinc.
- 38% of the DV for copper.
- 31% of the DV manganese.
- 13% of the DV for selenium.
- 39% of the DV for thiamin (vitamin B1).
- 5% of the DV for niacin (vitamin B3).
- 6% of the DV for vitamin B5.
- 8% of the DV for vitamin B6.
- 6% of the DV for folic acid (vitamin B9).

Flaxseeds are also rich in lutein and zeaxanthin, antioxidant phenolic compounds and flavonoids, and lignans, a type of polyphenol. You can also find small amounts (between 1 and 4%) of B-complex vitamins, vitamin E, vitamin K and choline in each ounce of flaxseeds. Parenthetically, most of these nutrients are not present in flaxseed oil. Flaxseed oil and capsules contain pure fat and lack most of the nutritional value that whole and ground flaxseed products contain (15).

When flaxseeds are eaten whole, for all intents and purposes they supply only the fiber and the lignans. In order to benefit from the omega-3 FA in the flaxseeds, however, the seeds must be chewed well or milled/ground. There is a number of sources where one can purchase organic whole flaxseeds online. For instance:

- Anthony's Organic Flaxseed Meal
- Essential Organics. ORGANIC FLAX SEEDS, golden
- Fesh Direct. Bob's Red Mill Organic Raw Whole Flaxseed
- FGO Whole Brown Flaxseed
- Great Origins. BROWN FLAX SEED—GROUND
- iHerb. Frontier Co-op, Organic Whole Flax Seed
- Nuts.com. Organic Flaxseed
- Premium Gold Whole Flax Seed
- Spectrum Essentials Organic Ground Premium
- Swanson Health Products. NOW Foods—Organic Flax Seed

Whole flaxseeds can be stored at room temperature for up to 10 months.

Alternatively, one may decide to grind or mill the whole flaxseed. Whole seeds can be ground at home using a coffee grinder, food processor or seed mill. A number of such devices are available for purchase online. For instance:

- COOL KNIGHT Herb Grinder Electric Spice Grinder (electric)
- Cuisinart SG-10 Electric Spice-and-Nut Grinder (electric)
- Glass Sesame Seed Grinder by Asvel (hand power)

Flax Is Good for You—At-Home Supplementation   125

- Mini Seed Mill & Coffee Grinder (electric)
- Staub Cast Iron Grinder (hand power)

There are approximately 1.6 g of omega-3 FAs in 1 tbsp of ground flaxseeds. When it is eaten ground/milled, all nutritional benefits, i.e., omega-3 FAs, fiber and lignans in the flaxseeds are preserved. Ground flaxseeds are best stored in the refrigerator or freezer and for no longer than 3 months. If one grinds the seeds, it is best to grind as needed, to prevent spoilage.

7.8 FLAX OIL

Flax oil is extracted from the whole flaxseed. It is sold as oil or in gel capsules. It is best to keep flax oil in a cool, dark place—ideally in the refrigerator. Flax oil is an excellent source of omega-3 FA, but it contains neither the lignans nor the fiber as these are eliminated in the process of oil extraction. A number of flax oil products are available including:

- Barlean's, Organic Fresh, Flax Oil
- Flax Oil. Radiant Life
- Flora, Certified Organic Flax Oil
- Puritan's Pride Organic Flaxseed Oil
- Solgar, Earth Source, Organic Flaxseed Oil

There is approximately 7.2 g of omega-3 FA in 1 tbsp of flax oil.
Capsules:

- Barlean's, Lignan Flax Oil
- Bluebonnet Nutrition, Organic Flax Seed Oil, 1,000 mg
- Jarrow Organic Flaxseed Oil (1,000 mg)
- Organic Flax Oil 1,000 mg—100 Soft Gels. Physician Naturals
- Solgar, Flaxseed Oil, 1,250 mg, 250 Softgels

These are just examples of what's available. There are many others, and the concentration, number of capsules per bottle, and prices vary. The manufacturers' best-before date tells us how to determine how long it can be stored. It is best to keep in mind that to obtain the benefits of the entire flaxseed, the best way to consume it is in the form of the ground (or milled) flaxseed/flax meal (16).

7.9 INCLUDING FLAXSEED IN DAILY DIET

One can:

- Add 1 tbsp of ground flaxseed to hot or cold breakfast cereal.
- Add 1 teaspoon (tsp) of ground flaxseed to mayonnaise or mustard when making a sandwich.

- Mix 1 tbsp of ground flaxseed into an 8 oz container of yogurt.
- Bake ground flaxseed into cookies, muffins, breads and other baked goods.

Like other sources of fiber, flaxseed should be taken with plenty of water or other fluids, and it shouldn't be taken at the same time as oral medications because the high fiber content might bind certain medications and thereby prevent their absorption.

One can also find a number of recipes online for including flaxseed in meals. The bullet point list that follows provides key words that can be entered into the online search field, but at the end of this section we do give the online source of most of these items:

- Flaxseed oatmeal, smoothies and yogurt bowls.
- Adding flaxseed to oatmeal, smoothies and yogurt bowls.
- Flaxseed and blueberry oatmeal.
- High-protein strawberry flax smoothie.
- Chia and flaxseed breakfast bowl.
- Apple pie overnight oats.
- Low-carb yogurt parfait with strawberries, flax and chia seeds.
- Flaxseed breads, tortillas, muffins and loaf recipes.
- Chia and flaxseed tortillas.
- Flax, carrot, apple muffins.
- Healthy oatmeal chocolate chip cookies.
- Flaxseed meal pancakes.
- Honey flax banana bread.

Flaxseed snack recipes:

- No-bake energy bites.
- Honey almond flax granola.
- Easy crunch flaxseed crackers.
- Flaxseed apricot bars.
- Power biscotti.

Other flaxseed recipes:

- Healthy baked turkey meatballs.
- Flaxseed chicken tenders.
- Almond flax crusted fish.
- Veggie-flax burgers.
- Keto low-carb meatballs.[1]
- TopTeenRecipes—16 Easy Flaxseed Recipes: https://topteenrecipes.com/flaxseed-recipes/.
- EatingWell— Healthy Flax Seed Recipes: https://www.eatingwell.com/recipes/19239/ingredients/nuts-seeds/flax-seed/.

- CookingLight—15 Ways to Use Ground Flaxseed: https://www.cookinglight.com/food/recipe-finder/ground-flaxseed-recipes.
- Profusion Curry—Flaxseed Garlic Chutney—Superfoods Chutney: https://profusioncurry.com/flaxseed-garlic-chutney-superfoods-chutney/tps://profusioncurry.com/flaxseed-garlic-chutney-superfoods-chutney/nutrition.
- Refined— Flaxseed Bread: https://nutritionrefined.com/flaxseed-bread/.

7.10 FLAXSEED RECIPE BOOKS

There are also books with flaxseed recipes, including:

Bakema M. 2015. *Flaxseed Recipes: Lose Weight, Gain Energy, & Achieve Overall Wellness.* CreateSpace Independent Publishing Platform.

Pitmon D. 2021. Recipes for Flaxseed: *Delicious Meal Recipes, How to Make Flaxseed for Breakfast, Soup, Smoothie, and More: Most Popular Flaxseed Recipes.* Independently published.

Bloomfield B., J. Brown and S. Gursche. 2000. *Flax the Super Food! Over 80 Delicious Recipes Using Flax Oil and Ground Flaxseed (Over 80 Delicious Recipes Using Flax Oil & Ground Flaxseed).* Kindle Edition. Book Publishing Company (TN).

Vincent E. 2013. *Flaxseed Recipes: How to Use Flaxseed in Omega 3, Low Carb, Wheat Free, Egg Free, Celiac Disease and Gluten Free Recipes. Includes 36 Flax Seed Recipes.* Kindle Edition. Sidewinder Media.

Niles S. 2014. *Flaxseed Recipes: 50 Delicious Recipes Using Flaxseed to Reduce Weight and Firing Up Your Metabolism Rate.* Paperback. CreateSpace Independent Publishing Platform.

7.11 CAVEAT

Finally, a word of caution: Flaxseed contains the vitamin B6 antagonist *linatine*. A clinical study published on the *Science.gc.ca* website concluded that daily consumption of 20–30 g of ground flaxseed can impair vitamin B6 status in adults who have elevated plasma levels of low-density lipoproteins (LDL). The study showed that the treatment regimen raised plasma homocysteine level, a marker of declining B6 (17). The study does not indicate that this outcome would also apply to individuals with normal LDL levels, but there is no reason to think that it might not do so. Epidemiologic evidence suggests that low dietary intake or reduced blood concentrations of vitamin B6 is associated with an increased risk of cardiovascular disease, although most recent trials demonstrated the ineffectiveness of vitamin B6 supplementation[*] on the prevention of cardiovascular events recurrence (18).

---

[*] Vitamin B6, pyridoxine, is not particularly well absorbed. Most sources recommend supplementing with a metabolite of the vitamin known as pyridoxal-5-phosphate, sometimes called P-5-P, because it is the active form of vitamin B6.

It might be a good idea to incorporate foods high in vitamin B6 in the diet when supplementing flaxseed. According to the Harvard School of Public Health website, these include:

- Beef liver.
- Tuna.
- Salmon.
- Fortified cereals.
- Chickpeas.
- Poultry.
- Some vegetables and fruits, especially dark leafy greens, bananas, papayas, oranges and cantaloupe (19).

NOTE

1. 25 Simple Flaxseed Recipes by Noom. September 20, 2019; Last updated February 15, 2022; https://web.noom.com/blog/25-simple-flaxseed-recipes/; accessed March 10, 2022).

REFERENCES

1. https://www.healthyflax.org/health/ask-expert.php; accessed 3/2/22.
2. https://www.mayoclinichealthsystem.org/hometown-health/speaking-of-health/flaxseed-is-nutritionally-powerful#:~:text=While%20there%20are%20no%20specific,2%20grams%20of%20dietary%20fiber; accessed 3/2/22.
3. https://www.livestrong.com/article/518919-how-much-flax-seed-oil-should-i-use-per-day/; accessed 3/2/22.
4. https://www.health.harvard.edu/heart-health/why-not-flaxseed-oil; accessed 3/2/22.
5. Calado A, Neves PM, Santos T, and P Ravasco. 2018. The effect of flaxseed in breast cancer: A literature review. *Frontiers in Nutrition*, 5: 4. DOI: 10.3389/fnut.2018.00004.
6. https://www.mountsinai.org/health-library/supplement/omega-3-fatty-acids#:~:text=Symptoms%20of%20omega%2D3%20fatty,fatty%20acid)%20in%20the%20diet; accessed 3/6/22
7. Thompson M, Hein N, Hanson C, Smith LM, Anderson-Berry A, Richter CK, Bisselou KS, Appiah AK, Kris-Etherton P, Skulas-Ray AC, and TM Nordgren. 2019. Omega-3 fatty acid intake by age, gender, and pregnancy status in the United States: National Health and Nutrition Examination Survey 2003–2014. *Nutrients*, Jan; 11(1): 177. DOI: 10.3390/nu11010177.
8. Patterson E, Wall R, Fitzgerald GF, Ross RP, and C Stanton. 2012. Health implications of high dietary omega-6 polyunsaturated fatty acids. *Journal of Nutrition and Metabolism*, 2012: 539426. DOI: 10.1155/2012/539426.
9. Parikh M, Maddaford TG, Austria A, Aliani M, Netticadan T, and GN Pierce. 2019. Dietary flaxseed as a strategy for improving human health. *Nutrients*, May; 11(5): 1171. DOI: 10.3390/nu11051171.
10. https://www.ncbi.nlm.nih.gov/books/NBK56068/table/summarytables.t4/?report=objectonly; accessed 3/9/22.
11. https://www.medicalnewstoday.com/articles/omega-6-fatty-acids#food-sources; accessed 3/9/22.

12. Surette ME, 2008. The science behind dietary omega-3 fatty acids. *Canadian Medical Association Journal (CMAJ)*, Jan 15; 178(2): 177–180. DOI: 10.1503/cmaj. 071356.
13. https://www.consumerreports.org/cro/news/2015/03/cost-of-organic-food/index.htm; accessed 3/9/22.
14. Sargi SC, Silva BC, Santos HMC, Montanher PF, Boeing JS, Santos OOJr, Souza NE, and JV Visentainer. 2013. Antioxidant capacity and chemical composition in seeds rich in omega-3: Chia, flax, and perilla. *Food Science and Technolology*, Sept; 33 (3). https://doi.org/10.1590/S0101-20612013005000057.
15. Healthline: https://www.healthline.com/ nutrition/foods/flaxseeds; accessed 3/12/21. https://www.mayoclinic.org/healthy-lifestyle/nutrition-and-healthy-eating/expert-answers/flaxseed/faq-20058354; accessed 4/12/21.
16. https://badgut.org/information-centre/a-z-digestive-topics/flax-what-you-need-to-know/; accessed 3/12/21.
17. Blewett HJ, Petkau J, Ren L, Guzman R, Wolever T, and M Aliani. 2018. Daily consumption of 20–30 g ground flaxseed impairs vitamin B-6 status in a randomized, controlled, crossover trial in adults with above-optimal plasma low-density lipoprotein concentrations (OR06-08). *Science.gc.ca*: https://profils-profiles.science .gc.ca/en/publication/daily-consumption-20-30-g-whole-ground-flaxseed-muffin-impairs-vitamin-b6-status; accessed 3/10/22.
18. Friso S, Lotto V, Corrocher R, and SW Choi. 2012. Vitamin B6 and cardiovascular disease. *Sub-Cellular Biochemistry*, 56: 265–290. DOI: 10.1007/978-94-007-2199-9_14.
19. https://www.hsph.harvard.edu/nutritionsource/vitamin-b6/; accessed 4/5/22.

8 Flax Is Good: Fish and Other Sea Critters Are Better

I know human beings and fish can co-exist peacefully.

—George W. Bush[*]

8.1 PHYTOPLANKTON 101

It all starts with plants: Fish are chuck-full of omegas, but fish don't actually make omegas. They eat fish that eat fish, that eat fish that eat critters that eat plants (microalgae, i.e., phytoplankton) that make omegas.

Derived from the Greek words *phyto* (plant) and *plankton* (made to wander or drift), phytoplankton are microscopic organisms that live in watery environments, both salty and fresh. Some of them are bacteria, some are protists, i.e., any organisms whose cells contain a nucleus but that are not animal, plant or fungus. Most phytoplankton are single-celled plants.

Phytoplankton have been around for nearly 3 billion years, and they are the basis of all life formed on earth. Transforming oxygen (O_2) into carbon dioxide (CO_2), they are responsible for creating the earth's atmosphere and allowing life to flourish. These powerful microalgae are bursting with all the nutrients needed to sustain life on the cellular level. Every life-giving molecule that makes up the entire planet can be found in different strains of marine phytoplankton. The nano-sized nutrient particles they make are easily absorbed and quickly ready to be used by the body.

Phytoplankton are extremely diverse. Like land plants, they have chlorophyll to capture sunlight, and they use photosynthesis to turn it into chemical energy, thus consuming carbon dioxide and releasing oxygen. But some of them get additional energy by consuming other organisms. Like land plants, they require nutrients such as nitrate, phosphate, silicate and calcium at various levels, depending on the species. They are the foundation of the aquatic food web depicted in Figure 8.1, the primary producers, feeding everything from microscopic animal-like zooplankton to multi-ton whales. Small fish and invertebrates also graze on the plant-like organisms, and then those smaller animals are eaten by bigger ones (1).

The aquatic food web illustrates the interdependence of phytoplankton, fish and marine mammals. The concentration of omega oils rises in the level of

---

[*] https://proverbicals.com/fish-proverbs.

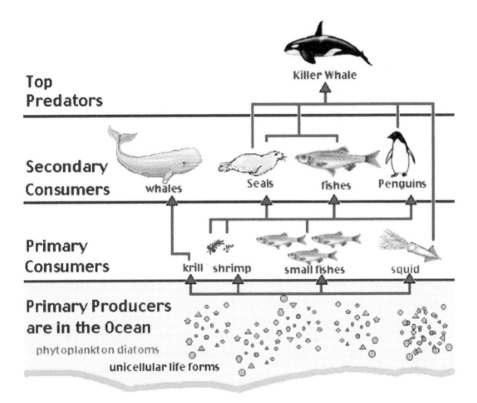

FIGURE 8.1 Plant plankton are eaten by krill, small crustaceans. Krill are eaten by fish; fish are eaten by seals and seals are eaten by whales. (From Alan S.L. Wong. https://www.pinterest.com/jeniferholly/ocean-food-web/. With permission.)

fish-eat-fish, up to marine mammal-predatory species. In fact, seal oil contains three omega-3 essential fatty acids (FAs): Docosapentaenoic acid (DPA), eicosapentaenoic acid (EPA) and docosahexaenoic acid (DHA), whereas fish oil contains only two: EPA and DHA. It is also better absorbed than fish oil (2). While it is generally illegal to import seal products into the United States, the Iñupiaq people in the Northwest Arctic (Alaska) have limited permission to do so (3). Also, harp seal oil—in capsules—from both Canada and the United States is available to American consumers:

- Seal Fat 500 milliliter (mL) eBay
- MapleLife Harp Seal Oil 1,000 milligram (mg) Omega-3
- Advanced Omega Newfoundland Omega-3 Original
- Herba Pure Canadian Harp Seal Omega-3, 500 mg

As might be expected, there is also a considerable amount of omega-3 and omega-6 FAs in blubber from bowhead whales. But this is unlikely to show up on a typical dinner plate or in supplement cabinets (4). By the way, we can bypass fish and go directly to the source—phytoplankton. For instance:

- Marine Phytoplankton Powder Raw Omega-3 EPA Vegan ATP Energy Superfood 100 grams (g); Longevity Herbs and Superfoods
- Marine Phytoplankton Nutritional Supplement Powder; Mr Ros Store
- Marine Phytoplankton Powder Capsules Raw Omega-3 EPA Vegan ATP Energy; Longevity Herbs and Superfoods
- Activation Products Oceans Alive Marine Phytoplankton—Pure Marine Phytoplankton Supplement Drops; Activation Products Store
- Sunfood, Ocean's Alive 2.0 Marine Phytoplankton

8.1.1 Caveat

We recommend that people seek advice on fish or other-source omega FA dosage supplementation from their healthcare provider. Excess omegas can be hazardous: As reported in the journal *Circulation* in 2021, Smidt Heart Institute researchers have found that taking high doses of the fish oil supplements EPA and DHA—specifically 1 g or more per day—may increase the risk of developing atrial fibrillation (5).

8.2 BUT BEFORE WE GET TO FISH …

Much in the previous chapters detailed omega-3s in flax and fish and their oils. This may have created the false impression that one can get omega-3s only from flax and fish. In fact, the omega-3 FAs have their origin in plant matter—land or sea-based plant matter. There are many other food sources—vegetable sources—from which one can get omega-3s. For instance:

- Broccoli—171 mg.
- Brussel sprouts—270 mg.
- Cabbage especially has 208 mg of omega-3 and just 62 mg of omega-6 per cup.
- Kale—120 mg, and it actually contains more omega-3 than omega-6, which is almost unheard of for its food type.
- Spinach—100 g of spinach contains 370 mg of omega-3.
- Soybeans—one bowl of lightly cooked soybeans contains more omega-3 than some cold-water fish, i.e., 510 mg per half cup serving.
- Winter squash has exceptionally high amounts of omega-3: 338 mg per cup (6).

Seaweed, by the way, can be an important source of omega-3 for people on a vegetarian or vegan diet as it is one of the few plant groups that contain both EPA and DHA. But the EPA and DHA contents vary depending on the type. For vegetarians and vegans, firm tofu, also plant derived, contains 582 mg/100 g, and avocado, 111 mg/100 g of omega-3 FAs.

The relatively high content of omega-3 FAs in many plant foods makes a strong case for the Mediterranean Diet. In fact, it is said that the Greek Mediterranean Diet—prior to the 1960s—had a ratio of total omega-6 to omega-3 FAs of about 2:1. In contrast, in the current diet of Greeks, the total ratio of omega-6 to omega-3 is about 10:1. This is closer to our Western diet, which can reach 15:1 or more (7).

However, of the three main types of omega-3 FAs, plant foods typically contain only alpha-linolenic acid (ALA). ALA is not as active in the body and must be converted to two other forms of omega-3 FAs—EPA and DHA—to bestow the same health benefits. EPA and DHA are plentiful in fish, and more fish is consumed in the Greek Mediterranean Diet than in the Western diets. That was pointed out in an earlier chapter in connection with the longer lifespan in Spain.

To know the omega-6:omega-3 ratio of a diet does not actually reveal how many omega-3s one consumes. To determine that, one would have to know the Omega-3 Index of people regularly on that particular diet. In fact, a study published in the journal *Nutrients* in 2021 aimed to determine whether the Mediterranean Diet, in comparison to a low-fat diet, favorably modifies the blood FA profile in patients with coronary heart disease on polytherapy, i.e., the use of two or more drug combinations with different mechanisms of action. Patients with a recent history of coronary stenting completed 3 months of this dietary intervention study.

Both diets significantly reduced saturated fats. However, favorable changes in total omega-3 FA and EPA + DHA were significantly larger with the Mediterranean Diet than with the low-fat diet. The investigators concluded that in these patients, the Mediterranean Diet more effectively shifts FA blood composition toward higher omega-3 levels (8).

What we learn from this study is that the Mediterranean Diet can raise the Omega-3 Index (which is desirable). But the study does not tell us that it can raise it enough to reach real health promoting levels, i.e., 8% or higher (9). However, a study published in 2011 in the *British Journal of Nutrition* reported that dietary data were obtained from Food Frequency Questionnaire (FFQ) and blood cell membrane FA composition from high cardiovascular risk participants on average 66 years old, living in Spain. Spain is noted for its low incidence of cardiac deaths despite a high prevalence of cardiovascular risk factors.

The investigators found that the average consumption of EPA + DHA was 0.9 g/day and the mean Omega-3 Index was 7.1%. EPA + DHA intake was the main predictor of the Omega-3 Index. However, they also concluded that the high Omega-3 Index could only partially explain the paradox of low rates of fatal coronary heart disease in Spain despite a high background prevalence of cardiovascular risk factors (10). There are a number of different regional Mediterranean Diets and there are other factors including genetic ones that are thought to also contribute to the impact of these diets on health and longevity.

The Mediterranean Diet does not include much red meat. Meat is usually high in omega-6 FAs, though grass-fed beef has a more favorable omega-6 to omega-3 FA ratio. While it is apparently the case that omega-6s *can* promote inflammation, in general, it is omega-6s in excess, compared to the intake of omega-3s that is problematic. Omega-6s are cardioprotective as previously shown, but in excess, compared to omega-3s, they actually inhibit the formation of omega-3s (from ALA) (11).

In any case, there is not just one type of Mediterranean Diet, and both the types of food and the quantities consumed in what is called "the Mediterranean Diet" actually vary considerably from region to region in the "Mediterranean" region. In addition, there is the issue of population compliance with the diet, region by region, as evaluated by the Mediterranean Diet Score (MDS).

8.3 THE MEDITERRANEAN DIET SCORE (MDS) VS THE OMEGA-6:3 RATIO

The MDS indicates compliance with the Mediterranean Diet. A high intake of Mediterranean foods, i.e., cereals, legumes, fruit, vegetables, fish, a high ratio of unsaturated FAs to saturated FAs, and wine, are scored positive (1) and a high intake of the non-Mediterranean foods such as dairy and meat are scored negative (0). The score can range from 0 to 9 and the higher the score the better the compliance to a traditional Mediterranean Diet. The website http://www.cardiacrehabilitation.org.uk/ docs/Mediterranean-Diet-Score.pdf offers a MEDITERRANEAN DIET SCORE TOOL intended for use by health professionals both as an audit tool and as part of a dietary assessment at baseline, end of program, and 1-year follow-up (12). In general, the MDS is inversely associated with the omega-6:3 ratio (7). What that means in plain English is that on a sound Mediterranean Diet with a high score, the omega-6s will tend to be lower and the omega-3s will tend to be higher, making for a low ratio of the two.

8.4 WHAT IS A FISH?

Officially, fish are completely aquatic vertebrates that have gills, scales and swim bladders to float. Most fish produce eggs, and are ectothermic, meaning cold-blooded. Sharks, stingrays, skates, eels, puffers, sardines and clownfish are all examples of fishes. Table 8.1 lists fish in accordance with the concentration of total omega-3 FA content and constituents, ALA, EPA and DHA.

Several popular fish were omitted from the chart. Sardines contain 982 mg of total omega-3s, three times as much as in farmed salmon at 230 g/100 g. And second, 100 g of arctic char has about 1.4 g of omega-3s per 100 g.

Sardines, part of the *Clupeidae* family which includes other small and oily fish like herring and anchovies, are small schooling fish that feed on plankton and small crustaceans. They are found in open oceans from Japan to California to Chile. They are called sardines after the island of Sardinia, an Italian Mediterranean island, where they were harvested in abundance. Sardines from different oceans have unique traits and subtle flavor differences, though once prepped, preserved in oil and canned, those nuances usually get lost. Also, before canning, sardines are often smoked or cooked by frying or boiling, so when the can is opened the fish is ready to eat. They may come packed in water, tomato juice or olive oil. Portugal is best known for sardines where they are a sort of national icon. Examples of readily available sardine products include:

- Numerous websites rank King Oscar Wild Caught Sardines in extra virgin olive oil as perhaps the best such product available commercially: https://www.kingoscar.com/product/brisling-sardines-in-extra-virgin-olive-oil/.
- The Spanish Martiz Gallego: https://www.matizespana.com/products/7seafood/7b_MatGal_sardines.html.
- Polar Sardines: https://www.mwpolar.net/sardines.
- El Manar: https://www.almanara.ca/products/sardines-el-manar-125g.
- La Brujula Sardinas: https://dibruno.com/la-brujula-sardines-in-olive-oil-31/.

According to the Cleveland Clinic website sardines provide a variety of benefits such as 2 g of heart-healthy omega-3s per 3-ounce (oz) serving, which is one of the highest amounts of omega-3s and the lowest levels of mercury of any fish. They are also a great source of calcium and vitamin D, so they support bone health, too (47).

TABLE 8.1
Omega-3 Fatty Acid Content of Fish

Species	Source	LNA* (18:3)	EPA* (20:5)	DHA* (22:6)	Total EPA + DHA	Total Ω-3 FAs	References
Lake Trout, Siscowet	freshwater	1.6	1.2	1.8	3.0	4.6	4
Mackerel, Atlantic	marine	0.1	0.9	1.6	2.5	26	2
Mackerel, King	marine	0.0	1.0	1.2	2.2	22	2,3
Dogfish, spiny	marine	0.1	0.7	1.2	1.9	2.0	2
Mackerel, Chub	marine	0.3	0.9	1.0	1.9	2.2	2
Salmon, Atlantic, farmed	marine	0.1	0.6	1.2	1.8	1.9	2
Herring, Pacific	marine	0.1	1.0	0.7	1.7	1.8	2,3
Herring, Atlantic	marine	0.1	0.7	0.9	1.6	1.7	2
Lake Trout	freshwater	0.4	0.5	1.1	1.6	2.0	2
Tuna, Bluefin	marine	0.0	0.4	1.2	1.6	1.6	2
Sturgeon, Atlantic	marine	trace	1.0	0.5	1.5	1.5	2
Chub	freshwater	1.1	0.7	0.8	1.5	2.6	4
Salmon, Chinook	both	0.1	0.8	0.6	1.4	1.5	2,3
Sablefish	marine	0.1	0.7	0.7	1.4	1.5	2
Anchovy, European	marine	0.0	0.5	0.9	1.4	1.4	2
Tuna, Albacore	marine	0.2	0.3	1.0	1.3	1.5	3
Lake Whitefish	freshwater	0.2	0.3	1.0	1.3	1.5	2
Sprat	marine	0.0	0.5	0.8	1.3	1.3	2
Trout, Lean Lake	freshwater	0.9	0.4	0.8	1.2	2.1	4
Salmon, Coho, farmed	both	0.1	0.4	0.8	1.2	1.3	2

(*Continued*)

TABLE 8.1 (CONTINUED)
Omega-3 Fatty Acid Content of Fish

Species	Source	LNA* (18:3)	EPA* (20:5)	DHA* (22:6)	Total EPA + DHA	Total Ω-3 FAs	References
Bluefish, Atlantic	marine	0.0	0.4	0.8	1.2	1.2	2,3
Herring, Round	freshwater	0.1	0.4	0.8	1.2	1.3	3
Salmon, Sockeye	both	0.1	0.5	0.7	1.2	1.3	2
Herring	freshwater	1.4	0.5	0.6	1.1	2.5	4
Capelin	marine	0.1	0.6	0.5	1.1	1.2	2
Whitefish	freshwater	0.8	0.5	0.5	1.0	1.8	4
Salmon, Pink	both	trace	0.4	0.6	1.0	1.0	2,3
Sardines, canned	marine	0.5	0.4	0.6	1.0	1.4	2
Salmon, Chum	both	0.1	0.4	0.6	1.0	1.1	2
Halibut, Greenland	marine	trace	0.5	0.4	0.9	0.9	3
Bass, Striped	freshwater	trace	0.2	0.6	0.8	0.8	3
Pompano, Florida	marine	0.0	0.2	0.4	0.6	0.6	3
Smelt	both	0.5	0.3	0.2	0.5	1.0	4
Mullet, Striped	both	0.1	0.3	0.2	0.5	0.6	3
Pollock	marine	0.0	0.1	0.4	0.5	0.5	3
Trout, Rainbow (Steelhead)	freshwater	0.1	0.1	0.4	0.5	0.6	3
Tuna, unspecified	marine	trace	0.1	0.4	0.5	0.5	3
Sucker	freshwater	0.2	0.2	0.2	0.4	0.6	4
Catfish, Brown Bullhead	freshwater	0.1	0.2	0.2	0.4	0.5	3
Halibut, Pacific	marine	0.1	0.1	0.3	0.4	0.5	3
Carp	freshwater	0.3	0.2	0.1	0.3	0.6	3
Catfish, Channel	freshwater	trace	0.1	0.2	0.3	0.3	3
Cod, Atlantic	marine	trace	0.1	0.2	0.3	0.3	3
Croaker, Atlantic	marine	trace	0.1	0.1	0.2	0.2	3
Flounder	marine	trace	0.1	0.1	0.2	0.2	3
Grouper, Red	marine	0.0	trace	0.2	0.2	0.2	3
Haddock	marine	trace	0.1	0.1	0.2	0.2	3
Perch, Ocean	marine	trace	0.1	0.1	0.2	0.2	3
Plaice, European	marine	trace	0.1	0.1	0.2	0.2	3
Snapper, Red	marine	trace	trace	0.2	0.2	0.2	3
Swordfish	marine	0.0	0.1	0.1	0.2	0.2	3
Burbot	freshwater	0.0	0.1	0.1	0.2	0.2	4
Sole, European	marine	trace	trace	0.1	0.1	0.1	3

Source: https://seafood.oregonstate.edu/sites/agscid7/files/snic/omega-3-content-in-fish.pdf; accessed March 16, 2022.

* g FA per 100 g of edible fish tissue or edible food.

* LNA is alpha-linolenic acid (ALA); EPA is eicosapentaenoic acid; DHA is docosahexaenoic acid.

References cited: 1: (15); 2: (16); 3: (17); 4: (18).

Herring deserves special mention. It has been a known staple food source since 3000 BCE In the Netherlands, herring has played a major role in historical and economic development dating back to the 14th century. Sometimes moving in vast schools, herring is caught, salted and smoked in great quantities. By the mid-13th century, herring had become one of the favorite foods in England.

The name "herring" refers to either the Atlantic herring (*Clupea harengus harengus*) or the Pacific herring (*C. harengus pallasii*). Herring is a small-headed, streamlined, beautifully colored fish with silvery iridescent sides and a deep blue, metallic-hued back. Adults range from 20 to 38 centimeters (cm) (8–15 inches (in)) in length. One of the most abundant species of fishes in the world, herring feed on minute organisms such as copepods, pteropods and other planktonic crustaceans, as well as fish larvae. It travels in vast schools, providing food for larger predators such as cod, salmon and tuna. In Europe the majority of the herring catch is either salted, pickled in barrels or cured by smoking and sold as kippered herring. In eastern Canada and the northeastern United States, most of the herring utilized are young fish canned as sardines. The bulk of the herring taken in the Pacific Ocean is used in the manufacture of fish oil and meal, and smaller quantities are pickled and smoked. Herring provides around 1.5 g of omega-3s per 3-oz serving which is more than is found in either salmon or tuna.

Atlantic herring is sometimes called a "kipper." This may have a historical basis because "kippering" is a form of preparation or "curing" by splitting it open and salting and drying it in the open air or in smoke. Herring is commercially available and some are still kippered:

- Bar Harbor Wild Herring Fillets, Cracked Pepper: https://barharborfoods.com/.
- MW Polar Herring, Kipper Snacks: https://www.mwpolar.net/kipper-herring.
- Brunswick Golden Smoked Herring Fillets: http://www.brunswicksardines.ca/ products/v/29.
- Season Peppered Kipper Snacks | Boneless Herring Fillets: http://www.season products.com/kippers/.
- King Oscar Kipper Snacks—Smoked Herring Fillets: https://www.kingoscar. com/products/kipper-snacks/.

Cod fish also does not appear in Table 8.1, perhaps due to its relatively modest omega-3s content but it is a relatively popular food. In the Northwest Atlantic, cod, one of the most popular food fishes in the Atlantic, ranges from Greenland to Cape Hatteras, North Carolina. In US waters, cod is most common on Georges Bank and in the western Gulf of Maine. Historically, cod was a favorite of European settlers as they learned to sustain themselves in North America. It can be recognized by its greenish-brown color and barbels (whiskers) on the chin. Cod contains about 221 mg of omega-3 FAs per 100 g, while the same serving of salmon contains 2,260 mg.

8.4.1 TILAPIA: BENEFITS AND CAUTIONS

Tilapia also does not appear in Table 8.1. It is an inexpensive, mild-flavored fish, the fourth most commonly consumed type of seafood in the United States. It is relatively affordable and doesn't taste very fishy, but, it has an undesirable omega-6:omega-3 ratio and several reports raise questions about tilapia farming practices in China and elsewhere overseas.

The name "tilapia" actually refers to several species of mostly freshwater fish that belong to the *Cichlid* family. Although wild tilapia is native to Africa, the fish has been introduced throughout the world and is now farmed in over 135 countries. China is by far the world's largest producer of tilapia providing the majority (73%) of US tilapia imports.

While tilapia is a good source of protein (3.5 oz/100 g), and vitamins and minerals (niacin, vitamin B12, phosphorus, selenium and potassium) as well as selenium (78% of the recommended dietary intake (RDI), see Section 8.18), it contains more omega-6 FAs than it does omega-3. According to research from Wake Forest University School of Medicine, ratios of long-chain omega-6 to long-chain omega-3, arachidonic acid (AA) to EPA, respectively, averaged about 11:1, compared to much less than 1:1 (indicating more EPA than AA) in both salmon and trout (47). The recommended ratio of omega-6 to omega-3 in the diet is typically as close to 1:1 as possible.

The website Healthline recommends that when shopping for farmed tilapia, the best sources are fish from the United States, Canada, the Netherlands, Ecuador or Peru (48). Some tilapia products imported from China and elsewhere were cited by the US Food and Drug Administration (FDA) for bacterial contamination (49).

8.5 HEALTH BENEFITS OF FISH

Fish have low-fat high-quality protein. They are full of omega-3 FAs and vitamins such as D and B2 (riboflavin). Fish is also rich in calcium and phosphorus, and it is a great source of minerals, such as iron, zinc, iodine, magnesium and potassium. The American Heart Association (AHA) recommends eating fish at least twice a week as part of a healthy diet because fish is packed with protein, vitamins and nutrients that can lower blood pressure and help reduce the risk of a heart attack or stroke.

8.6 COOKING FISH

Fish should be cooked to a minimum internal temperature of 145 degrees F (use a food thermometer to check) or until the meat is opaque and separates easily with a fork. Opaque means light can't pass through the fish meat and it no longer looks clear and shiny. The general cooking time for baking, poaching, broiling or grilling fish is about 10 minutes for every inch of thickness. For frozen, unthawed fish, double the cooking time to 20 minutes for every inch. Microwaving fish can significantly reduce cooking time. Follow package or recipe instructions to get the best results when cooking fish.

8.7 FISH—HOME DELIVERY

Fish can be purchased online, and it will be delivered virtually overnight from many vendors—fish farms and fisheries. For instance:

>Great Alaska Seafood
>720 Kalifornsky Beach Road
>Soldotna, Alaska 99669

Wild Salmon, Smoked Salmon, Giant Crab Legs, Colossal Scallops & Prawns from the Kenai Peninsula, Alaska. Their products can be ordered online: https://www.great-alaska-seafood.com/ and ordered by phone: 866 262-8846. They also offer recipes for seafood ranging from broiled or poached fish, crab, octopus and shellfish.

There are other vendors. For instance:

- KnowSeafood: https://knowseafood.com/.
- Butcher Box Seafood: https://www.butcherbox.com/shop/all-boxes/butcherbox-seafood-box?utm_source=affiliate&utm_medium=cpa&utm_term=389818&sscid=41k6_w7px.
- Island Creek Oysters: https://islandcreekoysters.com/.
- Luke's Lobsters: https://lukeslobster.com/collections/all-seafood.
- Pure Fish: https://www.purefish.com/?irclickid=V5Y1YnQrexyOUblwUx0Mo38OUkGQd-R5uXn4zE0&irgwc=1.
- Alaskan Salmon Co.: https://aksalmonco.com/?sscid=41k6_x43c&.

There are also many websites that offer fish and seafood recipes and cookbooks. For instance:

- D'Artagnan features fish and seafood recipes: https://www.dartagnan.com/seafood-recipes/?utm_medium=ppc&utm_ campaign=google-ads&utm_source=google&utm_content=search-ad&utm_term=&gclid=CjwKCAjwxZqSBhAHEiwASr9n9BAzexnBt61GbVdW8AHUVnJ7fIAYBgkz4wC8c65SQiczN770CgnzLBoCOQ4QAvD_BwE.
- America's Test Kitchen (Editor). 2020. *Foolproof Fish: Modern Recipes for Everyone, Everywhere*. America's Test Kitchen publisher.
- Hank Shaw. 2021. Hook, Line and Supper: New Techniques and Master Recipes for Everything Caught in Lakes, Rivers, Streams and Sea. H&H Books.
- Marine Stewardship Council. Sustainable Seafood Recipes: https://tinyurl.com/45ktzjxy.
- Fred Hutch. Cook for Life. 20 Easy Ways to Cook Fish This Week: https://tinyurl.com/24bcpf47.

8.8 FISH MAY HAVE CONTAMINANTS AND DANGEROUSLY HIGH LEVELS OF MERCURY

According to the Washington State Department of Health, to reduce exposure to contaminants remove the fish skin and visible fat before cooking. Grill, broil or bake the fish. Let the fat drip off during cooking. Avoid using the fat for gravy or sauces. See their fish fillet demonstration and get more tips on reducing exposure to contaminants in fish (17). Eat the fillet and no other parts and see Angler Wayne's Fish Fillet Demonstration (PDF): https://doh.wa.gov/sites/default/files/legacy/Documents/4300/ Fish-FilletDemo.pdf.

To reduce exposure to contaminants in fish, eat a variety of fish that are low in contaminants and see the *Healthy Fish Guide*: https://doh.wa.gov/community-and-environment/food/fish/healthy-fish-guide. *Check for local Fish Consumption Advisories*: https://doh.wa.gov/data-statistical-reports/washington-tracking-network-wtn/fish-advisories. Follow the *Statewide Mercury Advisories* for which fish to limit or avoid and advice on canned tuna: https://doh.wa.gov/community-and-environment/food/fish/ mercury-advisories. Eat smaller fish, they have fewer contaminants (18).

8.8.1 Concerning Mercury

Almost everyone has heard by now that we should limit our consumption of certain fish because they accumulate high levels of toxic mercury. Mercury, commonly known as *quicksilver*, is the only metal which is liquid at ordinary temperatures. It is poisonous. Natural activities such a forest fires and volcanic eruptions, and human industrial activities such as burning coal, oil and wood, send mercury into the atmosphere. Airborne mercury can fall to the ground in raindrops, in dust or simply due to gravity.

The amount of mercury deposited in a given area depends on how much mercury is released from local, regional, national and international sources. Once in a lake or river, mercury is converted to methylmercury by bacteria and other processes. Fish absorb methylmercury from their food and from water as it passes over their gills. Mercury is tightly bound to proteins in all fish tissue, including muscle.

As a general rule, smaller fish contain less mercury than larger varieties because when bigger fish eat smaller ones, they absorb their prey's contamination in a process known as *biomagnification*. So when a tuna eats anchovies, the tuna is accumulating the mercury of those anchovies in its own body.

The FDA provides a chart titled "Mercury Levels in Commercial Fish and Shellfish (1990–2012)," current as of February 25, 2022, sorted by MERCURY CONCENTRATION MEAN (PPM) from fish with the lowest levels of mercury to the highest levels of mercury: https://www.fda.gov/food/metals-and-your-food/mercury-levels-commercial-fish-and-shellfish-1990-2012. One can consult this chart for information on fish that we consume regularly. In general:

- King mackerel, marlin, orange roughy, shark, swordfish, tilefish, bluefish, ahi tuna and bigeye tuna all contain high levels of mercury. Women who are pregnant or nursing or who plan to become pregnant within a year should avoid eating these fish. So should children younger than 6. Tuna is the most common source of mercury exposure in the United States. If you or your kids regularly eat canned tuna, stick to light or skipjack tuna, and limit it to less than two servings a week. A 130-pound (lb) woman can eat almost two 6-oz

cans of light tuna a week and stay within the EPA-recommended safe zone for mercury. A 4- or 5-year-old child should eat only about 4 oz of light tuna per week. The rules change when it comes to albacore tuna. Children should avoid that fish altogether, and women of childbearing age should stick to no more than 4 oz per week.
- Popular sushi fish are often the apex predators of the food chain, so they tend to be high in mercury. If you are pregnant, nursing or planning a family, you can reduce mercury exposure from sushi by holding back on all types of tuna, mackerel, sea bass and yellowtail. Fish and shellfish like eel, salmon, crab and clam are lower in mercury.

These guidelines and many more can be found on the website of the *Natural Resources Defense Council* (NRDC), a US-based non-profit international environmental advocacy group: https://www.nrdc.org/stories/smart-seafood-buying-guide?gclid=Cj0KCQjwuMuRBhCJARIsAHXdnqNzK2LtIFqa-eVA0EDa5bzaieBcUzkELPVS pqh9YzbOQOb13Cc5UWEaAr1jEALw_wcB.

One of the main health benefits of fish is the omega-3 FAs they contain. But the amount of omega-3s varies considerably from type to type. Tilapia, and cod, for example, are all relatively low in omega-3 FAs. Whereas the best sources of omega-3s are salmon, sardines, sablefish, anchovies and herring. Among the shellfish, oysters are the only ones with comparable omega-3 levels (19).

8.9 SHELLFISH ARE NOT FISH

We distinguish between "seafood" and "shellfish": Seafood includes fish like tuna or cod, and shellfish like lobster or clams. In general, each type of seafood has its own unique nutritional profile, but we can also make some generalizations:

- All seafoods (with the exception of sea vegetables [seaweed]) are good sources of protein.
- Seafood is one of the better dietary sources of vitamin D.
- Mollusks tend to be rich in selenium and zinc.
- Crustaceans are often high in cholesterol.
- Because most seafood lives in salt water, they also are relatively high in sodium, compared with other animal proteins.

The following list compares omega-3 FA content in shellfish to that in salmon (20):

- Salmon (farmed):   2,252/3.0 oz
- Salmon (wild):   887/3.0 oz
- Shrimp: 267/3.0 oz
- Lobster: 71/3.0 oz
- Clams: 241/3.0 oz
- Oysters: 585/3.0 oz
- Crab: 351/3.0 oz

- Mussels: 665/3.0 oz
- Scallops: 310/3.0 oz

The standard serving size for any variety of meat or fish is 3 oz. Rather than weighing this out, the best visual indicator of this amount is roughly the size of the palm of your hand or the size of a standard deck of playing cards.

8.10 FISH OIL

*Web*MD recommends fish oil for heart health. According to its website, findings show omega-3 FA may help to lower cardiovascular risk. Concerning dosage, the AHA says that taking up to 3 g of fish oil daily in supplement form is considered safe, and not to take more than that unless one discusses it with one's doctor first (21). (Keep in mind the earlier caveat about atrial fibrillation.)

Healthline lists several benefits of supplementing with fish oil:

- *Improved cholesterol levels*. It can increase levels of high-density lipoprotein (HDL) (good) cholesterol and may also lower levels of low-density lipoprotein (LDL) (bad) cholesterol.
- *Decreased triglycerides*. It can lower triglycerides by 15–30%.
- *Reduced blood pressure*. Even in small doses, it helps reduce blood pressure in people with elevated levels.
- *Plaque prevention*. It may prevent the plaques that can cause arteries to harden, as well as make arterial plaques more stable and safer in those who already have them.

Dosage: Although EPA and DHA dosage recommendations vary according to age and health, for most adults, the World Health Organization (WHO) recommends a daily intake of 1.1–1.6 g (1,100–1,600 mg) of omega-3 FAs (22). That's about one tablespoon.

As summed up in a report by the Mayo Clinic, research on the use of fish oil has documented it to be effective in treating a variety of specific conditions, including:

- *Heart disease*: While research shows that people who eat dietary sources of oily fish at least twice a week have a lower risk of dying of heart disease, taking fish oil supplements seems (according to the report, which may be flawed in this respect) to have few if any benefits to heart health.[*]
- *High blood pressure*: Multiple studies report modest reductions in blood pressure in people who take fish oil supplements. There's some evidence that the beneficial effects of fish oil might be greater for people with moderate to severe high blood pressure than for those with only mild blood pressure elevation.

---

[*] This is a curious conclusion: "taking fish oil supplements seems to have little to no benefits to heart health" in light of the fact that, as they note, fish oil reduces triglycerides. Triglycerides are now considered an independent risk factor for coronary artery disease. When triglycerides are elevated, lipoprotein metabolism is altered, which increases risk of coronary artery disease (23).

- *High triglycerides and cholesterol*: There's strong evidence that omega-3 FAs can significantly reduce blood triglyceride levels. There also appears to be a slight increase in levels of HDL (or "good") cholesterol, although an increase in levels of LDL (or "bad") cholesterol was also observed.
- *Rheumatoid arthritis*: Studies suggest fish oil supplements might help reduce pain, improve morning stiffness and relieve joint tenderness in people with rheumatoid arthritis. While relief is often modest, it might be enough to reduce the need for anti-inflammatory medications.

The site recommends doctor supervision: Taking high doses of fish oil supplements might increase the risk of bleeding and possibly increase the risk of hemorrhagic stroke (24).

A number of fish oil supplements are available to consumers:

- Carlson Labs, Norwegian, "The Very Finest Fish Oil," Natural Lemon Flavor, 1,600 mg, 16.9 fluid ounces (fl oz) (500 mL).
- Bernard Jensen's Fish Oil from Iceland Unflavored 8 fl oz.
- Complete Human 100% Natural Fish Oil.
- Oslomega, Norwegian Omega-3 Fish Oil, Natural Lemon Flavor, 16.9 fl oz (500 mL).
- NOW Omega-3 Fish Oil Lemon Flavored 16.9 fl oz in capsules.
- Wild Alaskan Omega-3 Fish Oil—"Easy Swallow Minis 2× Double Strength" 630 mg EPA + DHA Natural Supplement 120 Mini Softgels.
- Nordic Naturals ProOmega-D, Lemon Flavor—1,280 mg Omega-3 + 1000 IU D3-60 Soft Gels—High-Potency Fish Oil—EPA & DHA—Brain, Eye, Heart, Joint, & Immune Health—Non-GMO.
- Dr Tobias TRIPLE STRENGTH OMEGA-3 FISH OIL.
- Live Conscious OmegaWell.
- Nature Made Fish Oil 1,200 mg Softgels.

[*Note*: We remind the reader that these products are listed here (and elsewhere in the book) for informational purposes only, as examples of what is available to consumers. We have no knowledge of, nor can we guarantee purity, quality or safety of these products. *Caveat emptor*: The authors have no commercial interest in any of the specific products mentioned in this book.]

8.10.1 A Note on Cod Liver Oil

Cod liver oil has been used for centuries to prevent rickets due to vitamin D deficiency. People living in northern Europe have long relied on cod liver oil as a vitamin D supplement during the winter months when sunlight is scarce. The oil is extracted from the liver of Atlantic cod and then filtered for purity. The leading producers of cod liver oil supplements now are northern countries like Norway and Iceland, and it can be found in most American supermarkets and health food stores.

Cod liver oil contains vitamin A, a vital nutrient for immune system function, cellular growth, eye health and reproduction. Even more so, cod liver oil's high vitamin D content is what distinguishes it from other fish oils. Scientists estimate that over a billion people worldwide are vitamin D deficient or insufficient. Vitamin D deficiency is linked to bone fractures in the elderly and abnormal brain development in offspring. It may also lead to the development of metabolic syndrome, which involves the combination of high blood pressure, high glucose levels and high blood-oxidized lipids. This can contribute to coronary heart disease, diabetes and cancer.

Cod liver oil also contains the omega-3 FA DHA, but less of it than is found in fish oil. Arctic cod liver oil has about 9% EPA and 14% DHA, whereas fish oil provides about 18% EPA and 12% DHA. But cod liver oil often has more vitamin A than you need because both vitamins A and D accumulate in fish liver. We are cautioned not to consume more than 1.5 mg of vitamin A per day. Cod liver oil is readily commercially available as canned cod liver, oil or in capsules (softgels). Here are a few examples:

- Dropi Extra-Virgin Cod Liver Oil Liquid or capsules: https://dropi.com/.
- Nordic Naturals—Arctic Cod Liver Oil: https://www.nordic.com/products/arctic-cod-liver-oil/?variant=39472186589368.
- Solgar—Cod Liver Oil, Vitamins A & D: https://www.solgar.com/products/cod-liver-oil-softgels-vitamin-a-d-supplement/.
- ICan Icelandic Cod Liver in Own Oil Flavor: https://ican.is/products/ King OscarCodLiver.
- Belveder Premium Wild Cod Liver in Own Oil from Iceland: https://www.pveuromarket.com/Belveder-Cod-Liver-120g-673538061760-9872/.

8.11 EELS

Eels are actually fish (albeit typically longer) and are flatter than snakes. As marine animals, and unlike reptiles, eels breathe underwater with their gills, and therefore cannot survive outside of water. The eel was once a common food item in the Western world due to its affordability and nutritional value. However, in recent times, declining reserves and sustainability concerns have decreased the availability (and increased the price) of these fish. For instance, eel reserves have fallen by approximately 5% per year for more than 50 years (25, 26). Despite this, efforts are underway to improve the sustainability of the fish.

Eels are used around the world in many different ways, and they feature in every sort of dish from grilled to sushi. They are a popular food in Japan where more than 70% of the global eel catch is consumed. Four countries are now responsible for the majority of global eel production, i.e., China, Japan, Korea and Taiwan. Japan is the predominant global producer (27).

There are two primary varieties of eel:

- Freshwater eels tend to live alongside the coast, in rivers and lakes. For those familiar with Japanese cuisine, this variety is known as "unagi."
- Saltwater eels live in ocean water and are also known by the Japanese name of "anago."

Eel tends to be low in mercury and offers a good amount of omega-3 (28):

- 838 mg omega-3 per 100-g serving (29).

If one is not into Kabayaki grilling, canned grilled eel can be purchased at:

- Instacart Broiled Eel Unagi Kabayaki
- Old Fisherman Roasted Eel, Black Bean, 3.5 oz (100 g)
- The Fresh Lobster Company Freshwater Charcoal Broiled Eel (9 oz) Unagi Kabayaki (Eel)
- HSIN TUNG YANG Roasted Eel in Sauce (Braised | Hot)
- eBay: Hamanako Shokuhin Unagi Kabayaki Grilled Eel 4 oz. Hard to find! Product of Japan

In addition, detailed eel food facts can be found at: https://fdc.nal.usda.gov/fdc-app.html#/food-details/174194/nutrients; accessed March 21, 2022.

8.12 FISH ROE/CAVIAR, SEA URCHIN AND SEAWEED

Per each 100 g of product, salmon roe contains 3.5 g of omega-3 FA, and caviar contains 6.8 g, which for the caviar would be approximately 1 tablespoon (tbsp) worth.

Fish roe and caviar are available to consumers at:

- ROYAL OSETRA CAVIAR (Tablespoon: 100 g [3.5 oz] $150.00)
- Wild Alaskan Keta Salmon Roe Ikura—2 oz jars 60402H
- Agustson Black Lumpfish Caviar Roe—12 oz
- Sam's Caviar: Pink Trout Roe Caviar, Pink Trout Ikura
- Catalina Offshore Products Tobiko Caviar (Flying Fish Roe)

Bottom line: Anyone can get omegas from just about everything that lives in or off the lakes, rivers or oceans.

A number of roe food products are common in what we call "sushi." Tobiko is Japanese for flying fish eggs, but the actual fish is found in the icy waters off Iceland. The flavor of the eggs is mild, which makes the perfect vehicle to infuse with pretty much any ingredient that adds color and flavor. It is usually found topping sushi rolls and nigiris, a familiar style of sushi made up of an oval-shaped mound of rice with a slice of raw fish on top.

Ikura is the Japanese term for salmon roe. It's sometimes called red caviar as well. These large eggs have a soft texture, a briny flavor and a mild fishiness. Ikura is also one of the healthier ingredients one can enjoy. Salmon roe is sourced in the late summer and fall from fish that are still in the ocean. The roe is typically brined in salt before being frozen at very cold temperatures. Soy sauce is sometimes substituted for brine. Either way, the salt and sub-zero freezing allow ikura to be available year-round.

Uni is the Japanese word for the edible part of the sea urchin and often used in nigiri sushi, sashimi or served with salad and pasta. Uni sushi is a staple in many Japanese restaurants.

The sea urchin contains 0.5 g of omega-3 FA per 100 g and, in addition, it also contains small amounts of anandamide, a lipid mediator that acts as an endogenous ligand of cannabinoid (CB1) receptors. These receptors are also the primary molecular target responsible for the pharmacological effects of Δ9-tetrahydrocannabinol, the psychoactive ingredient in *Cannabis sativa*.

Nori is the most recognizable seaweed. It usually comes pressed into thin dried sheets that are dark green or black, and which can be eaten as a snack or used to make sushi rolls. There are others including Wakame, Kombu, Dulse and Hijiki. Seaweed and algae are important sources of omega-3 for people on a vegetarian or vegan diet, as they are one of the few plant groups that contain both EPA and DHA.

Total omega-3 content per serving size:

- Nori: 4–134 mg/oz
- Wakame (kelp): 4–134 mg/oz

[*Note of caution to persons with diabetes*: We remind the reader that these foods are high in iodine and that iodine raises blood sugar.]

8.13 SHRIMP, PRAWN AND LOBSTER

Shrimps and prawns belong to different suborders although they are very similar in appearance and the terms, shrimps and prawns, are now often used interchangeably. However, we increasingly use the term "prawn" only for the freshwater forms and "shrimp" for the marine form.

Shrimps (or prawns) are also a good source of omega-3 FAs, 367 mg/3-oz serving, but they have high levels of cholesterol. They are the most popular seafood in the United States, but only a tiny fraction of that comes from domestic sources now. In fact, *caveat emptor*: 90% of the shrimp we eat is imported, and almost all of that comes from fish farms in Southeast Asia and Central America. A 3-oz (85-g) serving contains 166 mg of cholesterol. That's almost 85% more than the amount of cholesterol in other types of seafood, such as tuna.

It is common to fear foods that are high in cholesterol because we believe that they increase blood cholesterol and thus promote heart disease. However, this may not be the case for most people because only a small portion of the population is sensitive to dietary cholesterol. For the rest, dietary cholesterol may only have a small impact on blood cholesterol levels (30, 31). This is because most of the cholesterol in blood is produced by the liver, and when we eat foods high in cholesterol, our livers produce less of it (30, 31).

Shrimps and other seafood are also good sources of iodine because they absorb some of the iodine that is naturally present in seawater. Three ounces of shrimp contain about 35 micrograms (μg) of iodine, or 23% of the daily recommended intake. The recommended minimal daily intake of iodine to maintain a healthy thyroid and avoid hypothyroidism is 150 μg/day (250 μg /day for pregnant women). To avoid hyperthyroidism, we are advised not to exceed 600 μg/day. In terms of shrimp, that would be about 4 lb of shrimps each day.

8.13.1 KRILL AND KRILL OIL

Krill are small crustaceans of the order *Euphausiacea* found in all the world's oceans. They have been harvested as a food source for humans and domesticated animals since at least the 19th century and possibly earlier in Japan, where it is known as okiami. Large-scale harvesting of krill developed in the late 1960s and early 1970s, and now occurs only in Antarctic waters and in the seas around Japan. It is an uncommon food in the United States—understandably—as they are quite salty, and the hard exoskeleton must be removed before consuming them because it contains fluorine, which is toxic in high enough concentrations. However, krill oil is consumed here as a supplement, and it can be purchased online, usually in capsule form. For instance:

- KrillWell Heart, Joint and Cognitive Support | Certified Sustainable
- NOW Foods, Neptune Krill 1000, Double Strength, 1,000 mg
- NativePath Antarctic Krill Oil
- Swanson, 100% Pure Krill Oil
- Puritan's Pride Maximum Strength Red Krill Oil 1,500 mg

Krill oil contains the omega-3 FAs EPA and DHA. The chemical structure of its FAs and its red color set it apart from fish oil. Although krill oil is said to be "promising" in connection with cardiovascular function, and it offers the efficient delivery of omega-3 FAs in a smaller, more convenient capsule; nevertheless as of 2014 a report in the journal *Hospital Pharmacy* tells us, its benefits in that connection "remain unproven" (45).

Caveat: Krill oil, just like fish oil, can slow blood clotting and so it might increase the risk of bleeding in people with bleeding disorders, or people on anticoagulant medications. The same caution about food allergy also applies to krill as it does to shrimp.

8.14 SHELLFISH ALLERGY IS NOT LIKELY TO BE IODINE ALLERGY

According to the website FARE, Living with Food Allergies, shellfish allergies are the most common food allergies in adults and among the most common food allergies in children. Approximately 2% of the US population reports an allergy to shellfish, and these allergies are usually lifelong. When a person with an allergy to a particular shellfish is exposed to that shellfish, proteins in the shellfish bind to specific immunoglobulin E (IgE) antibodies made by their immune system. This triggers immune defenses leading to reaction symptoms that can range from mild to very severe.

There are two groups of shellfish: Crustaceans such as shrimp, prawn, crab and lobster; and mollusks/bivalves such as clam, mussel, oyster, scallop, octopus, squid, abalone and snail. Allergy to crustaceans is more common than allergy to mollusks, with shrimp being the most common shellfish allergen for both children and adults (32).

Some people have experienced an allergic reaction attributed to iodine in contrast material used for CT scans. The Mayo Clinic website reports that this is probably not an allergy to the iodine, as the thyroid gland in every person contains iodine. It is more likely that the allergic reaction is to the proteins in shellfish from which it is typically derived (33).

A number of websites offer recipes for shrimp/prawn:

- Healthy Shrimp Dinner Recipes: 8 Ways to Get More Omega-3s; https://spoonacular.com/articles/8-healthy-shrimp-dinner-recipes.
- Extra Virgin Olive Oil With Baked Shrimp & Veggies; https://morocco-gold.com/recipes/extra-virgin-olive-oil-with-baked-shrimp-veggies/.
- 15+ Easy, Healthy Shrimp Recipes: https://www.walderwellness.com/easy-healthy-shrimp-recipes/.
- Garlic Prawns (Shrimp): https://www.recipetineats.com/garlic-prawns-shrimp/.

Lobsters are large marine crustaceans, a type of shellfish. They have a long body with muscular tails and live in crevices or burrows on the sea floor. Three of their five pairs of legs have claws, including the first pair which are usually much larger than the others. Lobster is typically prepared by boiling or steaming. It can be eaten as a main course, enjoyed as sandwich filler or added to rich dishes like pasta, mashed potatoes and eggs Benedict.

To most folks in the Eastern United States and Canada, there is "only one kind of lobster," which is the American lobster, *Homarus americanus*. However, the scampi popular in Italy are also a type of lobster, and the more distantly related spiny lobsters popular in Australia and the "Balmain Bug" slipper lobsters popular in Asia and Australia are sold as lobster as well. The United States consumes the most American Lobsters, followed by Canada. Export markets of live American Lobsters go to Italy, Spain and France more than any other countries. Lobster supplies 0.25 g of omega-3 per 100-g serving. This amounts to 0.75 g of omega-3 per medium-sized lobster.

There are a number of ways to prepare lobster. For instance:

- Seven Heart-Friendly Lobster Recipes: https://www.healthline.com/health/high-cholesterol/lobster-recipes.
- THE BEST LOBSTER TAIL RECIPE EVER!: https://therecipecritic.com/lobster-tail-recipe/.
- Broiled Lobster Tails: https://vaya.in/recipes/details/broiled-lobster-tails/.
- 17 Dreamy Lobster Recipes to Master: https://www.foodandwine.com/seafood/shellfish/lobster/lobster?
- 10 Restaurant-Worthy Seafood Dishes to Cook at Home:[*] https://potatorolls.com/blog/10-restaurant-worthy-seafood-dishes/?gclid=Cj0KCQjw8_qRBhCXARIsAE2AtRZ47XVO3e8bnwQBjQYVkaPth9i5mgaw7dYmSBuTxVoNcqfNP9I2qyYaApDREALw_wcB.

It should be noted that all shellfish and crustaceans are high in cholesterol and iodine, and constitute, for some of us, a risk of mild to severe—even anaphylactic—allergic reaction. Furthermore, persons with Type 2 diabetes are cautioned to monitor their blood sugar levels more carefully when consuming foods high in iodine. As previously noted, iodine raises blood sugar.

---

[*] Crabs and scallops make up a very small portion of the typical American diet. There is 351 mg of omega-3 FAs in 3.0 oz of crabmeat, and 310 mg in 3.0 oz of scallops.

8.15 OCTOPUS AND SQUID

Octopus is a marine mollusk, a cephalopod, meaning "head foot" in Greek. A ring of eight equally long arms are merged with the head and surround it. The squid is also a cephalopod. It has a long, tapered body and eight short arms and two usually longer tentacles.

Octopus is commonly eaten in Hawaii, Korea, Japan and the Mediterranean, especially Spain, Portugal and Greece, where it is considered a delicacy. Squid is commonly served in Spain, China, Portugal, Greece, Taiwan and many other Asian and Mediterranean countries. According to the USDA Nutrient Database (2007), cooked octopus contains about 56 calories per 100 g and is a source of vitamin B3, B12, potassium, phosphorus and selenium.

8.15.1 Caveat

We are cautioned, however, that octopus heads are high in selenium and are also a risk for cadmium poisoning, even in small amounts. In 2010, more than 29 mg of cadmium was found in the head of octopus imported to South Korea from China. That is 14 times higher than the permitted level. Cadmium and lead concentrations were found to be elevated in squid harvested in Malaysian waters (34). People who eat at sushi bars might therefore be well-advised to decline the sushi chef's offer to serve slices of the head of the octopus, which is considered a delicacy.

Octopus features prominently in many cuisines:

- It is a common ingredient in Japanese cuisine, including sushi.
- Giant octopus, long arm octopus and webfoot octopus are a common food ingredient in Korean cuisine, where some small species are sometimes eaten raw as a novelty food (considered a dangerous practice here).
- *Miruhulee boava* is a Maldivian delicacy made of octopus tentacles braised in curry leaves, chili, garlic, cloves, onion, pepper and coconut oil.
- A common preparation technique in Greece involves classic Greek spices and seasonings, often including olive oil, garlic cloves, oregano, pepper and lemon juice. On the whole, octopus is considered a superb meze especially alongside ouzo.
- Octopus is a very common food in Spanish culture. In the Spanish region of Galicia, *polbo á feira* (market fair-style octopus) is a local delicacy. Restaurants which specialize or serve this dish are known as *pulperías*.
- In Portugal, octopus is eaten *à lagareiro* (olive oil miller style—roasted with potatoes, herbs, onion, garlic and olive oil), or stewed with rice (arroz de polvo), as well as breaded and then deep fried, with rice and beans.
- Seafood, including octopus, is used extensively in Tunisia, grilled, roasted, in couscous, pastas or chorbas.
- In Turkey, octopus salad (*ahtapot salatası*) is one of the most popular cold mezes served in fish restaurants along with eggplant. Grilled or as a casserole, it can also be prepared hot.

- Octopus is eaten regularly in Hawaii, where many popular dishes are Asian in origin. Locally known by their Hawaiian or Japanese names (*he'e* and *tako*, respectively).

In a popular preparation of squid, the squid is chopped, breaded and fried. This is the so-called calamari, though "calamari" can mean any squid eaten as food. By the way, fried calamari has more calories than most other preparations of calamari. The FA DHA is higher in squid than in other seafood. In addition, they contain astaxanthin antioxidants. Recipes include:

- Calamari—A source of omega-3: https://www.news24.com/health24/diet-and-nutrition/healthy-diets/calamari-a-source-of-omega-3-20131031.
- Healthy Puttanesca-Style Sauteed Squid: https://www.walderwellness.com/healthy-puttanesca-style-sauteed-squid/.
- Grilled Squid: https://eatwellenjoylife.com/grilled-squid/.
- Extra Virgin Olive & Sauteed Calamari: https://morocco-gold.com/recipes/sauteed-calamari-in-garlic-extra-virgin-olive-oil/.
- Squid & Chorizo Salad with Bitter Greens + Smoked Paprika Aioli: https://omnomally.com/2015/02/11/squid-chorizo-salad-with-bitter-greens-smoked-paprika-aioli/.

8.16 OYSTERS AND CLAMS

Oysters and clams are both bivalves, which is to say edible mollusks enclosed in a two-sided shell, and although they have a lot in common, there is plenty that sets these two delicacies apart. For starters, diners can identify an oyster from a clam based on appearance alone. Oysters have irregular shells, and clams have smooth shells. While both are commonly served in coastal communities, oysters are typically more sought after. The following other differences may explain why oysters tend to be more popular than clams.

While both clams and oysters taste fresh and salty, they each have unique flavors. Clams are known for having a briny and pungent taste, while oysters have a smooth and buttery taste. Oysters are rich in phosphorus, zinc and potassium, while clams offer iron, manganese, vitamin C and selenium. Regarding omega-3s, there is 241 mg per 3.0-oz serving in clams, and 585 mg per 3.0-oz serving in oysters.

8.17 SCALLOPS

Scallops, related to clams, mussels and oysters, are bivalves (having a two sided shell), like clams and oysters. The shells are held together by the adductor muscle which is the part of the scallop Americans typically eat. There are many varieties of scallop, but the most common is the small bay scallop, found in East Coast bays and estuaries, and the larger sea scallop, which exists in deep, cold waters on the ocean floor. Bay scallops are usually less expensive than sea scallops, especially when the sea scallops are very large. No matter the type, the scallops should be a pale pink or light beige color with a soft texture.

There is 310 mg of omega-3 FA in a 3-oz serving. Sample recipes include:

- Seared Scallops with Creamy Grits: https://www.thespruceeats.com/seared-sea-scallops-with-creamy-grits-3060674.
- Traditional French Scallops with Sage Cream: https://www.thespruceeats.com/seared-scallops-in-sage-cream-recipe-1375509.
- Bay Scallops with Garlic: https://www.thespruceeats.com/scallops-with-garlic-3060666.
- A Couple Cooks—12 Easy Scallop Recipes: https://www.acouplecooks.com/scallop-recipes/.
- Epicurious—29 Scallop Recipes for Restaurant-Worthy Dinners at Home: https://www.epicurious.com/recipes-menus/simple-scallop-recipes-gallery.

8.18   COVID-19—SHELLFISH TO THE RESCUE

WE ARE ABOUT TO CONVEY THAT RICH SOURCES OF A PARTICULAR NUTRIENT ARE PROTECTIVE AGAINST COVID. BEFORE PRESENTING THE SCIENTIFIC EVIDENCE UNDERLYING THAT POINT, WE WANT TO EMPHASIZE THAT THE FIRST LINE OF DEFENSE AGAINST COVID-19 MUST BE VACCINES, SOCIAL DISTANCING AND MASKS. Thus, the recommendation to strive to get adequate amounts of the particular nutrient in question must be understood in the context that it is NOT INSTEAD OF vaccines, masking and social distancing, but, rather, in addition to and synergistic with those sensible defenses.

There may be a better shot at avoiding Covid-19 infection, experiencing less severe symptoms—even avoiding dying from this disease—if one hails from a region of the world where soil selenium is plentiful, and it gets into the foods. There is scientific evidence that the trace mineral selenium found in the ground, plentiful also in shellfish, can lessen the risk of Covid infection, lessen the severity of the infection in those who contracted it, and reduce the risk of death from the infection. The evidence comes in part also from the increased risk in persons with low serum selenium levels, as well as from the lower risk in those in whom levels are normal or above normal through diet or supplementation.

An important clue to the role of selenium in connection with Covid-19 was first revealed in a study titled "Association between regional selenium status and reported outcome of COVID-19 cases in China," published in the *American Journal of Clinical Nutrition* in 2020. Apparently, there is a "belt of selenium deficiency" running from northeast to southwest in the country and, indeed, China has populations that have both the lowest and the highest selenium status in the world. Selenium deficiency results in insufficient antioxidant protection in viral infections.

The investigators collected real-time data from a non-governmental Chinese (People's Republic) website that provides daily updates of the reports of the health commissions of each province, municipality or city on numbers of Covid-19 confirmed cases, numbers cured and numbers who died. Selenium levels were based on hair concentration samples.

Hubei has abnormally low selenium levels in the soil and therefore in foods; and, accordingly, people from this area tend to have very low selenium levels in their tissues.

They found that the cure rate inside Hubei Province, of which Wuhan is the capital, was significantly lower than that in all other provinces combined (designated outside Hubei): a low cure rate of 13.2% in Hubei, compared with 40.6% outside Hubei.

Correspondingly, the death rate inside Hubei Province was significantly higher than the death rate in provinces outside Hubei: 3.0% compared with 0.6%, respectively. These analyses show that the outcome data for Hubei and outside Hubei are statistically distinct, separating Hubei (where mortality was much higher) and outside Hubei.

For instance, the cure rate in Enshi city, at 36.4%, was much higher than that of other Hubei cities, where the overall cure rate was 13.1%. The Enshi cure rate was significantly higher than that in the rest of Hubei Province. Enshi is renowned for its high selenium intake and status compared to typical levels in Hubei—so much so that selenium toxicity was actually observed there in the 1960s.

Similar data from provinces outside Hubei show that Heilongjiang Province in northeast China, a notoriously low-selenium region in which Keshan is located, had a much higher death rate than that of other provinces (35). The region of Keshan is of medical significance, because selenium levels are so low there that there has been widespread cardiomyopathy leading to heart failure. When it was discovered in the 1970s that the low selenium levels in the soil and in the food is the underlying cause of the cardiomyopathy, the disorder came to be called "Keshan Syndrome" (46).

According to *Web*MD, the recommended dietary allowance (RDA) for selenium is shown in Table 8.3.

The safe upper daily intake limit for selenium is 200 µg for adults. Anything above that is considered an overdose and may be toxic. The Mayo Clinic website tells us that the normal concentration in adult human blood serum is 70–150 nanograms (ng)/mL (0.15 parts per million) with a population mean value of 98 ng/mL (36).

Covid and Selenium Deficiency—The aim of a study titled "COVID-19 and selenium deficiency: a systematic review," published in the journal *Biological Trace Elements Research* in 2021, was to summarize the available data about the association of body selenium levels with the outcomes of Covid-19. The investigators found that in most cases, selenium levels in Covid-19 patients were lower than in healthy individuals and that selenium deficiency was associated with worse outcomes. And they concluded that selenium supplementation in Covid-19 patients may be helpful to prevent disease progression (37). Another team of investigators likewise published their conclusions in the same journal, in the same year, that decreased serum selenium levels may be a risk factor for the Covid-19 infection (38).

Selenium Deficiency Increases the Risk of Death from Covid—Because the risk of death from severe diseases like sepsis is inversely related to selenium status, investigators hypothesized that this finding might also apply to Covid-19. They reported in the journal *Nutrients*, in 2021, that serum samples from Covid-19 patients showed a pronounced deficit in total serum selenium. Furthermore, the selenium status was significantly higher in surviving Covid patients as compared to non-survivors, recovering with time in survivors while remaining low or even declining in non-survivors (39).

Selenium Supplementation Lessens the Severity of Covid—The purpose of this review published in the journal *Current Nutrition Reports* in 2021 was to determine how selenium status can modify the risk of Covid-19 infection, and how selenium

TABLE 8.2
Omega-3 Content per 4-oz Cooked Portion

Anchovies	Alaskan Pollock	Catfish	Cod
Herring	Barramundi	Clams	Crayfish
Mackerel (Atlantic & Pacific)	Crab	Flounder/Sole	Haddock
	Mussels	Grouper	Lobsters
Oysters (Pacific)	Salmon (Chum, Pink & Sockeye)	Halibut	Mahi Mahi
Sablefish (Black Cod)		Mackerel (King)	Shrimp
Salmon (Atlantic, Chinook, Coho)	Sea Bass	Perch	Scallops
	Squid	Rockfish	Tilapia
Sardines (Atlantic & Pacific)	Tilefish	Snapper	Tuna (Yellowfin)
	Tuna (Albacore/White)	Tuna (Skipjack)	
Swordfish			
Trout	Walleye		

Source: USDA National Nutrient Database for Standard Reference.

TABLE 8.3
Recommended Dietary Allowance (RDA) of Selenium

Group	Recommended Dietary Allowance
Children 1–3	20 micrograms/day
Children 4–8	30 micrograms/day
Children 9–13	40 micrograms/day
Adults and children 14 and up	55 micrograms/day
Pregnant women	60 micrograms/day
Breastfeeding women	70 micrograms/day

Source: https://www.webmd.com/a-to-z-guides/supplement-guide-selenium; accessed March 27, 2022 (45).

status might affect a person post-infection. It was found that selenium plays a key role in strengthening immunity, reducing oxidative stress, preventing viral infections and supporting critical illness. Moreover, selenium deficiency is related to hyper-inflammation seen in critical illness and with the severity of the disease. The investigators concluded that selenium supplementation at an appropriate dose may act as supportive therapy in Covid-19 (40).

Supplementing Sodium Selenite, not Selinate, Protects against Covid—According to a report published in the journal *Medical Hypotheses* in 2020, increased blood concentrations of selenium can be achieved with various pharmacological preparations, but only sodium selenite can offer true protection. Sodium selenite inhibits the entrance of viruses into the healthy cells and abolishes their infectivity. Therefore, this simple chemical compound can potentially be used in the battle against the current coronavirus epidemic (41).

In fact, CHRISTUS Health and Pharco Pharmaceuticals are co-conducting an interventional clinical trial (gov Identifier: NCT04869579) titled "Selenium as a potential treatment for moderately-ill, severely-ill, and critically-ill COVID-19 patients (SeCOVID)." Given its anti-viral, anti-oxidative, immune-enhancing, cytokine-modulating and anticoagulant properties, the investigators hypothesize that selenium infusion at supranutritional doses for moderately ill, severely ill and critically ill Covid-19 patients will prevent further clinical deterioration thus decreasing overall mortality and improving survival (https://clinicaltrials.gov/ct2/show/NCT04869579; accessed March 28, 2022).

One might consider occasionally consuming shellfish or supplementing selenium (with the approval of a healthcare provider, of course). For instance:

- Admart Healthvit Sodium Selenite Selenium 40 μg

or

- Douglas Laboratories Seleno-Methionine | 200 μg—Bioavailable Selenium
- Thorne Research—Selenomethionine—200 μg

8.19 JELLYFISH

Jellyfish (*Scyphozoans*) are not particularly popular food in the United States. However, they are widely consumed in Burma, China, Indonesia, Korea, Malaysia, the Philippines and Thailand. Jellyfish can be eaten in many ways including shredded or sliced thinly and tossed with sugar, soy sauce, oil and vinegar for a salad. It can also be cut into "noodles," boiled and served mixed with vegetables or meat. Jellyfish has a very delicate flavor, sometimes a bit salty. It's more about the texture, somewhere between a cucumber and a glass noodle, not as gelatinous as you might expect.

While low in fat, studies have shown that about half of the fat in jellyfish comes from polyunsaturated fatty acids (PUFAs) omega-3 (280 mg/100 g).

8.20 MUSSELS AND ABALONE

Mussel is the common name of several families of bivalve mollusks found in saltwater and freshwater habitats. These have a shell whose outline is elongated and asymmetrical compared with other edible clams, which are often more or less rounded or oval. Abalone are single-shelled snails with a large muscular foot that holds them to rocks. These two seafoods constitute only a very small portion of seafood consumed by Americans. For the record, mussels contain 665 g of omega-3 FAs per 3.0 oz; abalone contains only a tiny amount (49 mg) of DHA and EPA omega-3 FA/100 g. That's 0.002 oz.

8.21 CAVEAT

The University of Michigan Health—Michigan Medicine website informs us that eating raw shellfish, especially oysters, may put us at risk for hepatitis A. Bivalves such as oysters and clams filter large amounts of water when feeding. If shellfish are living in water that has been contaminated with stool containing the hepatitis A virus, the shellfish may carry the virus (42). The Center for Food Safety of the Government of Hong Kong Special Administrative Region offers the following advice:

- Buy only those shellfish which are fresh, with intact shell and free from abnormal odor.
- Do not buy shellfish from illegal hawkers and unlicensed food premises.
- Scrub and rinse the shellfish in clean water.
- All shellfish should be cooked at boiling temperature for not less than 5 minutes before eating.
- Mud oysters should not be eaten raw.
- If possible, remove the shells before cooking as they impede heat penetration.
- Remove the viscera of the shellfish before cooking.
- When having hotpot, use separate chopsticks and utensils for handling raw and cooked food to avoid cross contamination (43).

Finally: A word of caution in connection with regularly consuming omega-3 FAs from fish. A review of clinical studies (RCTs) examining cardiovascular outcomes, published in 2021 in the journal *Circulation*, reported that marine omega-3 supplementation was associated with an increased risk of atrial fibrillation. The risk appeared to be greater in trials testing more than 1,000 mg of EPA and/or DHA per day (44).

REFERENCES

1. https://earthobservatory.nasa.gov/features/Phytoplankton; accessed 3/21/22.
2. https://canadiansealproducts.com/blog/seal-oil-vs-fish-oil-5-reasons-seal-oil-always-wins; accessed 3/21/22.
3. https://www.alaskapublic.org/2021/02/01/it-brings-back-memories-northwest-alaska-health-provider-cleared-to-serve-seal-oil-to-elders/; accessed 3/21/.22.
4. Reynolds III JE, Wetzel DL, and TM O'Hara. 2006. Human health implications of omega-3 and omega-6 fatty acids in blubber of the bowhead whale (*Balaena mysticetus*). *Arctic*, 59(2): 155–164. DOI:10.14430/arctic338.
5. Gencer B, Djousse L, Al-Ramady OT, Cook NR, Manson JE, and CM Albert. 2021. Effect of long-term marine ω-3 fatty acids supplementation on the risk of atrial fibrillation in randomized controlled trials of cardiovascular outcomes: A systematic review and meta-analysis. *Circulation*, 144(25): 1981–1990. DOI: 10.1161/CIRCULATIONAHA.121.055654.
6. http://www.omega3benefit.com/blog/vegetables-omega3-fatty-acids; accessed 3/13/22.
7. Panagiotakos DB, Kastorini C-M, Pitsavos C, and C Stefanadis. 2011. The current Greek diet and the omega-6/omega-3 balance: The Mediterranean Diet Score is inversely associated with the omega-6/omega-3 ratio. In Simopoulos AP (ed): *Healthy Agriculture, Healthy Nutrition, Healthy People. World Review of Nutrition and Dietetics*, Basel, Karger, 102: 53–56. DOI: 10.1159/000327791.

8. Giroli MG, Werba JP, Risé P, Porro B, Sala A, Amato M, Tremoli E, Bonomi A, and F Veglia. 2021. Effects of Mediterranean Diet or low-fat diet on blood fatty acids in patients with coronary heart disease. A randomized intervention study. *Nutrients*, 13: 2389. DOI: 10.3390/nu13072389.
9. https://omegaquant.com/what-is-the-omega-3-index/; accessed 3/15/22.
10. Sala-Vila A, Harris WS, Cofán M, Pérez-Heras AM, Pintó X, Lamuela-Raventós RM, Covas M-I, Estruch R, and E Ros. 2011. Determinants of the Omega-3 Index in a Mediterranean population at increased risk for CHD. *British Journal of Nutrition*, 106(3): 425–431. DOI: 10.1017/S0007114511000171.
11. Román GC, Jackson RE, Gadhia R, Román AN, and J Reis. 2019. Mediterranean Diet: The role of long-chain ω-3 fatty acids in fish; polyphenols in fruits, vegetables, cereals, coffee, tea, cacao and wine; probiotics and vitamins in prevention of stroke, age-related cognitive decline, and Alzheimer disease. *Revue Neurologique (Paris)*, Dec; 175(10): 724–741. DOI: 10.1016/j.neurol.2019.08.005.
12. http://www.bacpr.com/resources/46C_BACPR_Standards_and_Core_Components_2012.pdf; accessed 3/13/22
13. Exler J. 1987. Composition of foods: Finfish and shellfish products. *Agriculture handbook 8–15*. Washington, DC: U.S. Dept. of Agriculture, Human Nutrition Information Service and Supt. of Docs., U.S. G.P.O.
14. Nettleton JA. 1995. *Omega-3 fatty acids and health*. New York: Chapman & Hall. pp. 21–30.
15. Spiller GA. 1996. *Lipid in human nutrition handbook, manuals*. Boca Raton: CRC Press. pp. 54.
16. Wang YJ, Miller LA, Ferren M, and PB Addis. 1990. Omega-3 fatty acid in Lake Superior fish. *Journal of Food Science*, 55(1): 71–73.
17. https://doh.wa.gov/about-us/programs-and-services/environmental-public-health/environmental-public-health-sciences/about-fish-advisories-program; accessed 3/21/22.
18. https://doh.wa.gov/community-and-environment/food/fish/reduce-contaminant-exposure; accessed 3/21/22.
19. https://www.verywellfit.com/the-best-fish-to-lose-weight-3495772; accessed 3/21/22.
20. Mozaffarian D, and EB Rimm. 2006. Fish intake, contaminants, and human health. Evaluating the risks and the benefits. *Journal of the American Medical Association (JAMA)*, Oct 18; 296(15): 1885–1899. DOI: 10.1001/jama.296.15.1885.
21. https://www.webmd.com/hypertension-high-blood-pressure/guide/omega-3-fish-oil-supplements-for-high-blood-pressure; accessed 3/21/22.
22. https://www.healthline.com/nutrition/benefits-of-fish-oil; accessed 3/21/22.
23. McBride P. 2008. Triglycerides and risk for coronary artery disease. *Current Atherosclerosis Reports*, Oct; 10(5): 386–390. DOI: 10.1007/s11883-008-0060-9.
24. https://www.mayoclinic.org/drugs-supplements-fish-oil/art-20364810; accessed 3/21/.22.
25. https://onlinelibrary.wiley.com/doi/full/10.1111/fme.12302; accessed 3/21/22.
26. https://www.ft.com/content/6acbbc1e-3588-11df-963f-00144feabdc0; accessed 3/21/22.
27. https://www.fao.org/fishery/en/culturedspecies/Anguilla_japonica/en; accessed 3/21/22.
28. https://fdc.nal.usda.gov/fdc-app.html#/food-details/174194/nutrients; accessed 3/21/22.
29. https://www.nutritionadvance.com/eel-nutritional-benefits/; accessed 3/21/22.
30. Fernandez ML, 2012. Rethinking dietary cholesterol. *Current Opinion in Clinical Nutrition and Metabolic Care*, Mar; 15(2): 117–121. DOI: 10.1097/MCO.0b013e32834d2259.
31. Berger S, Raman G, Vishwanathan R, Jacques P, and EJ Johnson. 2015. Dietary cholesterol and cardiovascular disease: A systematic review and meta-analysis. *American Journal of Clinical Nutrition*, Aug; 102(2): 276–294. DOI: 10.3945/ajcn.114.100305.

32. https://www.foodallergy.org/living-food-allergies/food-allergy-essentials/common-allergens/shellfish#:~:text=If%20you%20have%20a%20shellfish%20allergy%2C%20you%20do%20not%20need,in%20some%20radiographic%20medical%20procedures; accessed 3/26/22.
33. https://www.mayoclinic.org/diseases-conditions/shellfish-allergy/symptoms-causes/syc-20377503; accessed 3/25/22.
34. Jamil T, Lias K, Norsila D, and NS Syafinaz. 2014. Assessment of heavy metal contamination in squid (Loligo SPP) tissues of Kedah-Perlis waters, Malaysia. *Malaysian Journal of Analytical Sciences*, 18(1): 195 –203.
35. Zhang J, Taylor EW, Bennett K, Saad R, and MP Rayman. 2020. Association between regional selenium status and reported outcome of COVID-19 cases in China. *American Journal of Clinical Nutrition*, Jun 1; 111(6):1297–1299. DOI: 10.1093/ ajcn/nqaa095.
36. https://www.mayocliniclabs.com/test-catalog/overview/9765#:~:text=The%20normal%20concentration%20in%20adult,circulating%20selenium%20than%20do%20adults; accessed 3/27/22.
37. Fakhrolmobasheri M, Mazaheri-Tehrani S, Kieliszek M, Zeinalian M, Abbasi M, Karimi F, and AM Mozafari. 2021. COVID-19 and selenium deficiency: A systematic review. *Biological Trace Elements Research*, Nov; 5: 1–12. DOI: 10.1007/s12011-021-02997-4.
38. Younesian O, Khodabakhshi B, Abdolahi N, Norouzi A, Behnampour N, Hosseinzadeh S, Alarzi SSH, and H Joshaghani. 2022. Decreased serum selenium levels of COVID-19 patients in comparison with healthy individuals. *Biological Trace Elements Research*, Apr; 200(4): 1562–1567. DOI: 10.1007/s12011-021-02797-w.
39. Moghaddam A, Heller RA, Sun Q, Seelig J, Cherkezov A, Seibert L, Hackler J, Seemann P, Diegmann J, Pilz M, Bachmann M, Minich WB, and L Schomburg. 2020. Selenium deficiency is associated with mortality risk from COVID-19. *Nutrients*, Jul 16; 12(7): 2098. DOI: 10.3390/nu12072098.
40. Khatiwada S, and A Subedi. 2021. A mechanistic link between selenium and coronavirus disease 2019 (COVID-19). *Current Nutrition Reports*, Jun; 10(2): 125–136. DOI: 10.1007/s13668-021-00354-4.
41. Kieliszek M, and B Lipinski. 2020. Selenium supplementation in the prevention of coronavirus infections (COVID-19). *Medical Hypotheses*, Oct; 143: 109878. DOI: 10.1016/j.mehy.2020.109878.
42. https://www.uofmhealth.org/health-library/hw123919#:~:text=Eating%20raw%20shellfish%2C%20especially%20oysters,shellfish%20may%20carry%20the%20virus; ACCESSED 3/27/22.
43. https://www.cfs.gov.hk/english/programme/programmerafs/programme_rafs_fm_02_06.html; accessed 3/27/22.
44. Gencer B, Djousse L, Al-Ramady OT, Cook NR, Manson JE, and CM Albert. 2021. Effect of long-term marine ω-3 fatty acids supplementation on the risk of atrial fibrillation in randomized controlled trials of cardiovascular outcomes: A systematic review and meta-analysis. *Circulation*, 144(25): 1981–1990. DOI: 10.1161/CIRCULATIONAHA.121.055654.
45. Backes JM, and PA Howard. 2014. Krill oil for cardiovascular risk prevention: Is it for real? *Hospital Pharmacy*, Nov; 49(10); 907–912. DOI: 10.1310/hpj4910-907.
46. Shi Y, Yang W, Tang X, Yan Q, Cai X, and F Wu. 2021. Keshan disease: A potentially fatal endemic cardiomyopathy in remote mountains of China. *Frontiers in Pediatrics*, 9: 576916. DOI: 10.3389/fped.2021.576916.
47. Chilton FH, Weaver KL, Ivester P, Chilton JA, Wilson MD, and P Pandey. 2008. Popular fish, tilapia, contains potentially dangerous fatty acid combination. *ScienceDaily*, 10 July. <www.sciencedaily.com/releases/2008/07/080708092228.htm>.
48. https://www.healthline.com/nutrition/tilapia-fish.
49. https://www.accessdata.fda.gov/cms_ia/importalert_49.html.

9 Omega-3 Target and Six-Day Meals Plan

9.1 BEFORE YOU HEAD FOR THE KITCHEN

We have assembled a flexible, demonstration six-day meal plan with recipes that supply ample omega-3 fatty acids (FAs). We provide six breakfast, six lunch and six dinner meal recipes, and they can be arranged in any way that is suitable to taste. Periodically testing for the Omega-3 Index level is a good idea to determine the progress and success of the diet plan.

As noted in a previous chapter, Dr W.S. Harris, a pioneer in the development of the Omega-3 Index (O3I) (https://omegaquant.com/about/), suggests that

> people wait to retest for 4 months, the time it takes for red blood cells, on which the test is based, to all be replaced. One may, however, certainly see a rise in the Omega-3 Index (O3I) by 1 month, more at 2, etc. until at 4 months one is pretty close to being in a new steady state. [By his calculations,] if a person starts at 4% O3I, it will take 1200–1500 mg of additional EPA+DHA per day to get to 8% on average. Some people need more; others less, but that's a good starting point. With permission.

We suggest that one take the test at the start, at https://omegaquant.com/omega-3-index-basic/, and then retest at a later date.

In order to determine whether one is on the right track, there are information sources—food charts—that will tell us what we need to know about omega-3 concentrations in foods, which can be consulted when beginning a new omega-3-rich food plan.

9.2 OMEGA-3 INDEX TARGET: 8.0%

In planning daily meals, keep in mind that most authorities recommend a minimum of 250–500 milligrams (mg) combined eicosapentaenoic acid (EPA) and docosahexaenoic acid (DHA) each day for healthy adults (1–3). The recommended dietary allowance (RDA) for alpha-linolenic acid (ALA) is 1.6 grams (g) per day for men, and 1.1 g per day for women (4).

The Mayo Clinic recommendations are that:

- Adults should eat at least 8 ounces (oz) or two servings of omega-3-rich fish a week. A serving size is 4 oz or about the size of a deck of cards.
- Women who are pregnant, plan to become pregnant or are nursing should eat up to 12 oz of seafood per week from a variety of choices that are lower in mercury contamination.

- Children should also eat fish from choices lower in mercury, once or twice a week. The serving size for children younger than age 2 is 1 oz and increases with age (5).

*Web*MD recommends 500 mg daily of EPA + DHA, and people with known heart disease or heart failure should aim for nearly twice that amount (at least 800–1,000 mg daily) (6).

Between 2017 and 2019, the American Heart Association (AHA) released three science advisories on omega-3s (7–9). All three advisories recommend one to two servings of seafood per week to reduce the risk of heart disease and sudden cardiac death, especially when the seafood replaces foods that are less healthy (8). For people with existing coronary heart disease, such as a recent myocardial infarction, the AHA recommends approximately 1 g/day EPA plus DHA, preferably from oily fish; however, supplements could also be considered (under the direction of a physician) (7).

To achieve the recommended Omega-3 Index of 8.0%, one can calculate the EPA + DHA content of the foods chosen for any given meal by accessing that information on the following websites that provide ALA, DHA or EPA from the Office of Dietary Supplements Health Professional Fact Sheet on Omega-3 Fatty Acids:

Alpha-linolenic acid (ALA)

- https://ods.od.nih.gov/pubs/usdandb/ALA-Food.pdf; for instance: #05735. Turkey, retail parts, wing, meat and skin, cooked, roasted 85.0 g/3.0 oz, 0.173 g ALA.

Docosahexaenoic acid (DHA)

- https://ods.od.nih.gov/pubs/usdandb/DHA-Content.pdf; for instance: #15237. Fish, salmon, Atlantic, farmed, cooked, dry heat. 85.0 g/3 oz, 1.238 g DHA.

    [Note: The example shown by the Office of Dietary Supplements used farmed salmon, but for health reasons we would recommend that whenever possible (and affordable), wild-caught salmon would be preferable.]

Eicosapentaenoic acid (EPA)

- https://ods.od.nih.gov/pubs/usdandb/EPA-Content.pdf; for instance: #15165. Mollusks, mussel, blue, cooked, moist heat. 85 g/3oz, 0.430 gEPA.

The *NutritionData* website (https:// nutritiondata.self.com/foods-009140000000141 000000.html?maxCount=138; accessed January 23, 2022) lists "Foods Highest in Total Omega-3 Fatty Acids, and Lowest in Total Omega-6 Fatty Acids."

9.3 SOME PLANT SOURCES OF OMEGA-3 FATTY ACIDS

Omega-3s are not found only in flax and fish, but also in plant/vegetable foods. The following sites provide a list of good plant sources of omega-3 FAs.

- https://www.healthline.com/nutrition/7-plant-sources-of-omega-3s.

Omega-3-rich vegetarian foods: Vegetables, fruits and nuts

- https://www.wellcurve.in/blog/omega-3-vegetarian-foods-vegetables-fruits/.

Keep in mind also that omega-6 FAs are not harmful per se. In fact, many of them, such as nuts, are heart protective. Foods that are high in omega-6 FAs include:

- Walnuts: 10.8 g per 1-oz serving
- Grapeseed oil: 9.5 g per tablespoon (tbsp)
- Pine nuts: 9.3 g per 28-g serving
- Sunflower seeds: 9.3 g per 1-oz serving
- Sunflower oil: 8.9 g per tbsp
- Corn oil: 7.3 g per tbsp
- Walnut oil: 7.2 g per tbsp
- Cottonseed oil: 7.0 g per tbsp
- Soybean oil: 6.9 g per tbsp
- Mayonnaise: 5.4 g per tbsp
- Almonds: 3.7 g per 1-oz serving
- Tofu: 3.0 g per half cup
- Vegetable shortening: 3.4 g per tbsp

The website *NutritionData* provides a comprehensive list of foods ranked by omega-6 FA content: https://nutritiondata.self.com/foods-000141000000000000000-w.html (accessed March 23, 2022). In these categories:

- Cereal Grains and Pasta
- Breakfast Cereals
- Baked Products
- Vegetables and Vegetable Products
- Nut and Seed Products
- Legumes and Legume Products
- Finfish and Shellfish Products
- Poultry Products
- Beef Products
- Pork Products
- Lamb, Veal and Game Products
- Sausages and Luncheon Meats
- Dairy and Egg Products
- Soups, Sauces and Gravies
- Fats and Oils
- Snacks
- Sweets
- Spices and Herbs
- Baby Foods
- Ethnic Foods
- Fast Foods, Generic

The simplest way to determine the omega-3 or 6 content of any food per serving is the *NutritionData.Self* website.

Finally, there is a free app called "My Plate." To create a personal plan, or to track foods and nutrients eaten, the USDA provides a free interactive tool called SuperTracker at:

- https://www.choosemyplate.gov/resources/MyPlatePlan

9.4 HOW TO DETERMINE THE OMEGA-3 FATTY ACID COMPOSITION OF MEALS

Unless the omega-3 FA is from a marine source, it is likely to be ALA. Only about 5% of the ALA we eat gets converted to EPA, and of that, <1% goes on to produce DHA. The typical US intake of ALA is ~1,500 mg per day, so that would generate about 75 mg of EPA and <1 mg of DHA (10).

9.4.1 Some Sources of Omega-3-Rich Recipes

There are many websites that feature wonderful recipes for meals said to be rich in omega-3s as well as useful related products and advice on meal preparation. Here is a small sample of them:

- My Everyday Table—Back to School: Omega-3s for Breakfast. https://myeverydaytable.com/back-school-omega-3s-breakfast/.
- Omega-3s for Breakfast—Starting the day off right: http://www.omega-3benefit.com/blog/omega3s-for-breakfast-starting-day-off-right.
- *Web*MD—Ideas for Omega-3 Foods, Morning to Night: https://www.webmd.com/cholesterol-management/morning-night-guide-omega-3-foods.
- Bon Appétit—20 Recipes Full of Omega-3 Fatty Acids: https://www.bonappetit.com/recipes/healthy/slideshow/omega-3-recipes.
- Food Network—Omega-3-Rich Recipes: Omega-3-Rich Recipes (Guess What? They're Not All Fish).
- VegFAQS—15 Delicious Vegan Recipes High in Omega-3: https://vegfaqs.com/15-delicious-vegan-recipes-high-in-omega-3/.
- OneGreenPlanet—10 Healthy Vegan Omega-3-Rich Recipes: https://www.onegreenplanet.org/vegan-food/healthy-vegan-omega-3-rich-recipes/.
- EatingWell—8 Best Vegan Omega-3 Rich Foods: https://www.eatingwell.com/article/291962/8-best-vegan-omega-3-rich-foods/.

We have chosen some representative recipes to make up the six-day meals plan to give you an idea of how relatively simple it is to make healthy omega-rich meals. But you can look at some of the sources of recipes online and make your own choices. That said, *Bon Appétit*!

9.5 BREAKFAST RECIPES

9.5.1 Hearty Oatmeal Pancakes with Flax and Chia Seeds

You will need the following ingredients

- 3 cups gluten-free organic old-fashioned rolled oats divided (325 g).
- 2 teaspoon (tsp) baking powder (8 g).
- 1 tsp baking soda (4 g).

1 tsp kosher salt (6 g).
2 tbsp organic chia seed (25 g).
2 tbsp organic golden flaxseed meal (15 g).
¼ cup maple syrup (60 milliliters (mL)).
1 egg (50 g).
1 tsp vanilla extract (5 g).
1½ cups milk (360 mL).
2 tbsp butter for skillet (30 g).

Preparation instructions

Preheat a griddle or nonstick pan to medium heat.
Blend 2 cups of rolled oats in flour in a high-powered blender or food processor, about 30 seconds.
To the oat flour, add in baking powder, baking soda, salt, chia seeds and flaxseeds. Pulse to combine.
Add in the remaining cup of rolled oats, maple syrup, egg, vanilla extract and milk. Blend for 30–45 seconds or until combined and no dry spots remain.
Brush preheated griddle with butter and portion batter using a ¼ measuring cup. Cook until the edges begin to set, 3–4 minutes. Flip and continue to cook on the second side 2–3 minutes more. Serve warm or hold in a 200 °F oven for up to 15 minutes.

There are many other great recipes on the website: https://www.bobsredmill.com/recipes/how-to-make/hearty-oatmeal-pancakes-with-flax-and-chia-seeds/ (accessed April 12, 2022).

9.5.2 Blueberry Omega-3 Breakfast Bowl

You will need the following ingredients

- ½ cup gluten free quick oats.
- ½ cup frozen wild blueberries.
- 1 tbsp hemp hearts.
- 1 tbsp chia seeds.
- 1 tbsp unsweetened shredded coconut.
- 4 whole walnuts.
- 1 cup unsweetened oat milk.
- ½ tsp ground cinnamon.
- 1 tbsp honey.

Preparation instructions

Assemble oats, blueberries, chia seeds, hemp hearts, coconut and walnuts into a cereal bowl.

Top with oat milk, cinnamon and honey and stir. Let sit for 5 minutes to allow the oats to soak.

There are many other great recipes on the website: https://blastfitness.ca/blog/2020/02/23/blueberry-omega-3-breakfast-bowl/ (accessed April 12, 2022).

9.5.3 Homemade Açaí Bowl

You will need the following ingredients

- 7 oz frozen açaí puree.
- 1 cup almond milk.
- 1 frozen banana.
- 1 tbsp honey (optional).
- *Toppings*: Sliced fruit, berries, granola, peanut butter, etc. (See whole list of ideas above.)

Preparation instructions

Blend together açaí, milk, banana and honey.
Pour into bowls and top with desired toppings.

You will find many other great recipes on the website: https://myeverydaytable.com/classic-acai-bowl/#tasty-recipes-18675-jump-target (accessed April 12, 2022).

9.5.4 Mini Blueberry Muffin Recipe

You will need the following ingredients

- ¾ cup all-purpose flour.
- ½ cup whole wheat flour.
- ¼ cup old-fashioned oatmeal.
- ⅓ cup sugar.
- 1 tsp baking powder.
- ½ tsp baking soda.
- ½ tsp sea salt.
- ⅓ cup milk.
- ½ cup vanilla Greek yogurt.
- ½ cup melted butter.
- 1 large egg.
- 1 tsp vanilla.
- ½ cup blueberries + 1 tbsp flour (flour is for frozen blueberries).
- 1 tbsp coarse sugar (you may have extra).

Preparation instructions

Preheat oven to 425 °F.

In a large bowl, stir together all-purpose flour, whole wheat flour, oatmeal, sugar, baking powder, baking soda and sea salt.

In a medium bowl, whisk together milk, butter, eggs and vanilla until smooth.

Stir wet ingredients into dry ingredients and stir just until combined, being careful to not over mix. Fold in blueberries gently.

Divide mixture into mini muffin tin and bake for 7 minutes, then lower heat to 350 °F and bake for 6–8 more minutes, or until a toothpick inserted in the middle of a muffin comes out clean.

You will find many other great recipes on the website: https://myeveryday-table.com/mini-blueberry-muffins-recipe/#tasty-recipes-29536-jump-target (accessed April 12, 2022).

9.5.5 Greek Muffin-Tin Omelets with Feta and Peppers

You will need the following ingredients:

- Cooking spray.
- 2 tbsp extra virgin olive oil.
- ¾ cup diced onion.
- ¼ tsp salt, divided.
- 1 medium red bell pepper, diced.
- 1 tbsp finely chopped fresh oregano.
- 8 large eggs.
- ¾ cup crumbled feta cheese.
- ½ cup low-fat milk.
- ½ tsp ground pepper.
- 2 cups chopped fresh spinach.
- ¼ cup sliced Kalamata olives.

Preparation instructions

Preheat oven to 325 °F. Liberally coat a 12-cup muffin tin with cooking spray.

Heat oil in a large skillet over medium heat. Add onion and ⅛ tsp salt; cook, stirring, until starting to soften, about 3 minutes. Add bell pepper and oregano; cook, stirring, until the vegetables are tender and starting to brown, 4–5 minutes more. Remove from heat and let cool for 5 minutes.

Whisk eggs, feta, milk, pepper and the remaining ⅛ tsp salt in a large bowl. Stir in spinach, olives and the vegetable mixture. Divide among the prepared muffin cups.

Bake until firm to the touch, about 25 minutes. Let it stand for 5 minutes before removing from the tin.

Tips—To make ahead: Prepare through Step 3 and refrigerate egg mixture overnight. Let it stand at room temperature for 10 minutes before baking. The cooked omelets (wrapped individually in plastic wrap) can be refrigerated for up to 3 days or frozen for up to 1 month. To reheat, thaw, if necessary, and remove plastic wrap. Wrap in a paper towel and microwave each omelet on High for 20–30 seconds.

You will find many other great recipes on the website: https://www.eatingwell.com/recipe/277641/greek-muffin-tin-omelets-with-feta-peppers/ (accessed April 12, 2022).

9.5.6 MEDITERRANEAN TOFU SCRAMBLE

You will need the following ingredients

- 7 oz firm tofu.
- ½ tsp extra virgin olive oil.
- ¼ cup chopped red pepper.
- 2 cups baby kale and arugula blend.
- ⅛ cup thinly sliced red onion.
- ¼ cup cherry tomatoes.
- ¼ cup crumbled feta cheese.
- 1 tsp chopped chives.
- 2 tsp chopped flat-leaf parsley.
- Salt.
- Freshly ground pepper.

Preparation instructions

Place tofu on paper towels on a plate. Add paper towels on top of the tofu and place a cast iron skillet on top for 10 minutes to drain additional water.

Heat a medium skillet on the stove over medium-high heat. Add olive oil and red pepper. Sauté for 3 minutes. Add pressed tofu to the skillet and break up with a spoon to create a crumble. Add to a plate with greens. Top with tomatoes, feta, chives and parsley. Season with salt and pepper to taste.

There are many other great recipes on the website: https://www.eatthis.com/a-10-minute-mediterranean-tofu-scramble-recipe/ (accessed April 12, 2022).

9.6 LUNCH RECIPES

9.6.1 Mediterranean Shrimp Quinoa Bowl Recipe

You will need the following ingredients

- 1½ cups quinoa.
- 1 pound (lb) raw shrimp.
- ¼ cup olive oil.
- ¼ cup lemon juice (about one lemon).
- 1 large tsp of Dijon mustard.
- 1 tbsp oregano.
- ½ tsp salt.
- Pepper to taste.
- 12 oz jar roasted red peppers.
- 1 medium cucumber.
- 5 oz bag of herb salad mix.
- 4–6 oz feta cheese crumbles.

Preparation instructions

Prepare quinoa according to package instructions.
Thaw shrimp if necessary.
In a small jar combine olive oil, lemon juice, mustard, oregano, salt and pepper. Shake until combined.
Prep veggies: Drain red peppers and thinly slice. Wash and thinly slice cucumber. Wash lettuce if necessary.
Heat a large nonstick skillet over medium-high heat. When hot, add 2 tbsp of dressing to pan, along with shrimp. Cook for about 2–3 minutes, until shrimp is cooked through, careful to not overcook. (You'll know it's done when it turns pink and curls up.)
Assemble shrimp quinoa bowls: Divide quinoa in bowls and top with vegetables, shrimp and feta cheese. Drizzle with dressing.

There are also many other great recipes on the website: https://myeverydaytable.com/mediterranean-quinoa-bowls-with-shrimp/#tasty-recipes-17650-jump-target (accessed April 13, 2022).

9.6.2 Mexican Sardine Salad Stuffed Avocados

You will need the following ingredients

- 2 large avocados, halved and pit removed.
- 1 container Season Brand sardines, drained and rinsed.

- 1 bell pepper, finely diced.
- 1 Roma tomato, finely diced.
- ⅓ cup frozen corn.
- 1 green onion, diced.
- ½ lime, juiced.
- 1 tbsp olive oil.
- ¼ tsp cayenne powder.
- ½ tsp chili powder.
- ½ tsp cumin.
- 1 tsp garlic powder.

Preparation instructions

Mash the sardines with a fork. Mix together the rest of the ingredients besides the avocado.

Stuff the salad in the avocado. There will be extra salad that can't fit into the avocado so you can serve it on the side.

You will also find many other great recipes on the website: https://www.nutritionistreviews.com/2018/04/mexican-sardine-salad-stuffed-avocados.html (accessed April 13, 2022).

9.6.3 Salmon Cakes with Creamy Ginger-Sesame Sauce

You will need the following ingredients

- 6 slices whole-wheat sandwich bread.
- 2 (15-oz) cans salmon, drained, skin and bones removed.
- 2 eggs, lightly beaten.
- 5 scallions.
- ½ cup finely chopped canned water chestnuts.
- ¼ cup finely chopped fresh cilantro leaves.
- ½ tsp freshly ground black pepper.
- 3 tsp olive oil, divided.

Preparation instructions

Remove crusts from the bread, break into pieces and process in a food processor until you get a fine bread crumb. In a large bowl, flake apart the salmon with a fork. Add the egg and mix well. Finely chop 4 of the scallions and add to the bowl. Add the water chestnuts, cilantro, pepper and the breadcrumbs and mix well. Shape the mixture into 12 patties.

In a large nonstick skillet, heat 1½ tsp of olive oil over a medium heat. Add 6 patties and cook for 5 minutes on each side. Transfer the cooked patties to a plate and cover with foil to keep warm. Add the remaining 1½ tsp olive oil to the pan, and cook the rest of the salmon cakes, 5 minutes on each side.

Chop the remaining scallion. Serve salmon cakes with the sauce and garnish with scallion.

Creamy Ginger-Sesame Sauce:

- ½ cup non-fat plain yogurt, or 6 tbsp non-fat Greek-style yogurt.
- 2 tbsp mayonnaise.
- 1½ tbsp freshly grated ginger.
- 1 tsp toasted sesame oil.
- 1 tsp low-sodium soy sauce.

If using regular yogurt place the yogurt in a strainer lined with a paper towel. Put the strainer over a bowl and place in the refrigerator to drain and thicken for 30 minutes.

Place drained yogurt or Greek-style yogurt into a small bowl. Add mayonnaise, ginger, sesame oil and soy sauce. Whisk until smooth.

There are also many other great recipes on the website: https://www.foodnetwork.com/recipes/ellie-krieger/salmon-cakes-with-creamy-ginger-sesame-sauce-recipe-1947036 (accessed April 13, 2022).

9.6.4 Tuna and Green Bean Salad

You will need the following ingredients

- 1½ lb slender green beans, trimmed, halved crosswise.
- 3 tsp salt, plus more to taste.
- 2 large red potatoes, diced.
- ⅓ cup freshly squeezed lemon juice.
- 2 garlic cloves, finely chopped.
- ⅓ cup extra virgin olive oil.
- 1 tsp dried oregano.
- ¾ tsp freshly ground black pepper.
- 8 oz cherry tomatoes, halved.
- ½ cup chopped fresh basil leaves.
- ¼ cup chopped fresh Italian parsley leaves.
- 9 oz canned tuna packed in oil, drained.

Preparation instructions

Cook the green beans in a large pot of boiling water until crisp-tender, stirring occasionally, about 4 minutes. Using a mesh strainer, transfer the green beans to a large bowl of ice water to cool completely. Drain the green beans and pat dry with a towel.

Add 2 tsp of salt to the same cooking liquid and bring the liquid to a simmer. Add the potatoes to the simmering liquid and cook until they are just tender but still hold their shape, about 8–10 minutes. Transfer the potatoes to the ice water to cool completely. Drain the potatoes and pat dry with a towel.

In a small bowl, whisk the lemon juice, garlic, oil, oregano, 1 tsp salt and ¾ tsp pepper. Place the tomatoes, basil and parsley in a large serving bowl. Add the tuna and toss gently to combine. Add the green beans and potatoes and gently combine. Pour the dressing over the salad and toss to coat.

There are many other great recipes on the website: https://www.foodnetwork.com/recipes/giada-de-laurentiis/tuna-and-green-bean-salad-recipe-1916510 (accessed April 13, 2022).

9.6.5 Spinach Salad with Winter Squash and Walnuts

You will need the following ingredients

- 1 butternut (or other winter) squash, peeled and seeded, cut into 1-inch cubes (about 4 cups).
- 5 tbsp olive oil.
- 1¼ tsp salt.
- 8 oz spinach.
- 2 tbsp fresh-squeezed lemon juice.
- ½ tsp Dijon mustard.
- ⅔ cup walnuts.

Preparation instructions

Preheat oven to 450 °F. Toss squash with 1 tbsp olive oil to coat, season with 1 tsp salt, and spread in a single layer on a baking sheet. Bake, stirring after 20 minutes, until tender and lightly browned, about 30 minutes total. Add to a bowl with the spinach. Combine lemon juice, remaining 4 tbsp olive oil, mustard, and remaining ¼ tsp salt in a jar and shake vigorously, or whisk in a bowl until emulsified. Toss dressing with squash and spinach, and top with the walnuts. Tip: For texture and added health benefits, add 1 tsp chia seeds to the dressing.

There are also many other great recipes on the website: https://www.mensjournal.com/food-drink/guilt-free-omega-3-meal-plan/3-the-lunch-spinach-salad-with-winter-squash-and-walnuts/ (accessed April 13, 2022).

9.6.6 Grilled Sauerkraut Avocado Sandwich

You will need the following ingredients

- 8 slices pumpernickel bread.
- Vegan buttery spread (or regular butter).
- 1 cup hummus (roasted garlic flavor, divided).

- 1 cup sauerkraut (drained, lightly rinsed and liquid squeezed out).
- Avocado peeled and sliced lengthwise into about 16 pieces.

Preparation instructions

Preheat oven to 450 °F.

Spread butter on one side of each of the 8 slices of bread, and place 4 of them butter side down on a baking sheet.

Take about half of the hummus and distribute over the 4 slices of bread.

Distribute the sauerkraut over the hummus on each slice.

Distribute the avocado slices over the sauerkraut.

For the remaining 4 slices of bread, spread hummus on the side without butter and place hummus side down on the avocado slices.

Bake in the oven for 6–8 minutes, then flip the sandwiches and bake about 6 minutes more, until the sandwiches are golden brown and crispy. (Alternatively, you can grill them on the stove top on a griddle or in a skillet.)

You will also find many other great recipes on the website: https://dizzybusyand-hungry.com/moms-grilled-sauerkraut-avocado-sandwich (accessed April 13, 2022).

9.7 DINNER RECIPES

9.7.1 Green Tea Poached Salmon with Ginger Lime Sauce

You will need the following ingredients

- 10 cups water.
- 2 limes, halved.
- 6 tbs honey, divided.
- 4-inch piece fresh ginger, peeled and chopped.
- 2 tsp sea salt.
- 2 tsp whole black peppercorns.
- 4–6 tbsp loose green tea.
- 4 (6 oz) boneless skinless salmon fillets.

Preparation instructions

Put the water into a straight-sided skillet or pot with a lid. Add three of the lime halves (squeezing the juice into the water before adding), 5 tbsp of the honey, the ginger, salt and peppercorns and bring to a boil over medium-high heat. Reduce the heat to a simmer, cover, and cook for 10 minutes to infuse the water with flavors. Remove and reserve ½ cup of this poaching liquid. Remove the pot from heat and add the tea. Allow the tea to steep for 3–5 minutes. Carefully slide the salmon into the water. Cover and poach until the fish is just cooked through and firm to the touch, about 6–7 minutes.

Meanwhile, in a small pot over low heat, simmer the reserved ½ cup of liquid along with the juice and zest of the remaining lime half, and remaining

1 tbsp of honey. Cook until the liquid is reduced by ⅔ and thickened, 7–10 minutes.

Remove the fish with a slatted spoon and arrange on serving plates. Drizzle a little bit of the sauce over each piece of salmon before serving.

There are also many other great recipes on the website: https://www.foodnetwork.com/recipes/claire-robinson/green-tea-poached-salmon-with-ginger-lime-sauce-recipe-1922941 (accessed April 13, 2022).

9.7.2 Baked Mediterranean Fish Recipe

You will need the following ingredients

- 2 tbsp olive oil.
- 1 clove garlic, sliced.
- 16 cherry tomatoes, halved.
- 8 Kalamata olives, pitted and roughly chopped.
- 1 tbsp capers.
- Sea salt and pepper, to taste.
- 4–6 oz fillets flaky white fish.
- 1 small lemon, thinly sliced.
- 4 tbsp white wine.
- 1 small bunch basil, leaves torn.

Preparation instructions

Preheat oven to 400°F. Cut four large squares of parchment paper.

In a skillet over medium heat, add 1 tbsp oil. Add the garlic, tomatoes, olives and capers.

Sauté for 3 minutes, or until the ingredients begin to soften. Season with salt and pepper and set aside.

Place a fish fillet in the center of each piece of parchment. Arrange a lemon slice on top of each fillet and evenly divide the tomatoes, olives and capers among the fish parcels. Sprinkle with a pinch of sea salt and pepper. Drizzle with 1 tsp olive oil and 1 tbsp white wine.

Wrap each parcel by folding the sides together and creating a tent, ensuring there are no gaps as you fold the paper together.

Place the parcels on a baking sheet and bake for 8–10 minutes, or until the fish flakes easily and the flesh is opaque. Sprinkle the opened parcels with basil leaves and serve immediately.

You will also find many other great recipes on the website: https://myeverydaytable.com/steamed-mediterranean-fish-parcels/#tasty-recipes-17122-jump-target (accessed April 13, 2022).

9.7.3 SIMPLY POACHED SALMON

You will need the following ingredients

- 2 carrots.
- 1 celery stalk.
- 1 small onion.
- ½ lemon.
- Coarse salt.
- 4 skinless salmon fillets.

Preparation instructions

In a large, deep, straight-sided skillet or heavy pot, combine carrots, celery, onion, lemon, 1½ tsp salt and 6 cups water. Bring to a boil; reduce to a simmer, cover, and cook for 8 minutes.

Season salmon with salt and gently lower into simmering liquid (liquid should just cover fish). Reduce to a very gentle simmer. Cover and cook until salmon is opaque throughout, about 5 minutes (longer for thicker fillets). Using a wide slotted spatula, remove salmon from liquid.

There are also many other great recipes on the website: https://www.delish.com/cooking/recipe-ideas/recipes/a21642/simple-poached-salmon-recipe-mslo0114/ (accessed April 13, 2022).

9.7.4 SALMON SALAD WITH PARSLEY AND CAPERS

You will need the following ingredients

- ½ small red onion.
- 2 tbsp red wine vinegar.
- 3 tbsp chopped capers.
- 2 tbsp olive oil.
- ½ tsp coarse salt.
- 3 fillets simply poached salmon.
- ½ cup fresh parsley.

Preparation instructions

In a large bowl, combine red onion, red wine vinegar, capers, olive oil and salt. Let it stand for 10 minutes. Add salmon and parsley.

There are also many other great recipes on the website: https://www.delish.com/cooking/recipe-ideas/recipes/a22326/salmon-salad-parsley-capers-recipe-mslo0114/ (accessed April 13, 2022).

9.7.5 SLOW-ROASTED SALMON WITH FENNEL, CITRUS AND CHILES

You will need the following ingredients

- 1 medium fennel bulb, thinly sliced.
- 1 blood or navel orange, very thinly sliced, seeds removed.
- 1 Meyer or regular lemon, very thinly sliced, seeds removed.
- 1 red Fresno chili or jalapeño, with seeds, thinly sliced.
- 4 sprigs dill, plus more for serving.
- Kosher salt and coarsely ground black pepper.
- ½ lb skinless salmon fillet, preferably center-cut.
- ¾ cup olive oil.
- Flaky sea salt (such as Maldon).

Preparation instructions

Preheat oven to 275 °F. Toss fennel, orange slices, lemon slices, chili and 4 dill sprigs in a shallow 3-quart baking dish; season with kosher salt and pepper. Season salmon with kosher salt and place on top of fennel mixture. Pour oil over.

Roast until salmon is just cooked through (the tip of a knife will slide through easily and flesh will be slightly opaque), 30–40 minutes for medium-rare.

Transfer salmon to a platter, breaking it into large pieces as you go. Spoon fennel mixture and oil from baking dish over; discard dill sprigs. Season with sea salt and pepper and top with fresh dill sprigs. You can also try it with cod, halibut, John Dory or turbot fillets.

There are many other great recipes on the website: https://www.bonappetit.com/recipe/slow-roasted-salmon-with-fennel-citrus-and-chiles (accessed April 13, 2022).

9.7.6 HARVEST SQUASH MEDLEY

You will need the following ingredients

- 6 cups water.
- 1 butternut squash, peeled, seeded and cut into ¾-inch pieces.
- 2 medium sweet potatoes, peeled and cut into ¾-inch pieces.
- ¼ cup honey.
- ¼ cup orange juice.
- 3 tbsp butter.
- 1 tbsp grated orange zest.
- ½ tsp ground cinnamon.
- ⅛ tsp ground nutmeg.
- 2 small apples, peeled and sliced.
- ½ cup chopped walnuts, toasted.

Preparation instructions

In a large saucepan, bring water to a boil. Add squash and return to a boil. Reduce heat; cover and simmer for 10 minutes. Drain. Place squash and sweet potatoes in a greased 13 × 9-inch baking dish.

In a small saucepan, combine the honey, orange juice, butter, orange zest, cinnamon and nutmeg. Bring to a boil, stirring constantly. Pour over squash and potatoes.

Cover and bake at 350 °F for 30 minutes, stirring occasionally. Uncover; stir in apples. Bake 30–35 minutes longer or until tender, stirring occasionally. Sprinkle with walnuts.

You will also find many other great recipes on the website: https://www.tasteofhome.com/recipes/harvest-squash-medley/ (accessed April 13, 2022).

9.8 OPTIONAL DESSERTS

A number of omega-3-rich desert and smoothie recipes are available online:

- Grain Free Omega-3 Fudgy Walnut Skillet Brownies: https://www.ambitious kitchen.com/grain-free-omega-3-fudgy-walnut-skillet-brownies/.
- Omega-3 No-Bake Bars: http://nwhealthymama.com/2017/03/omega-3-no-bake-bars/.
- Chia Berry Parfait: https://unchainedtv.com/2021/03/26/healthy-dessert-mixed-berry-chia-parfait-and-pudding-recipes/
- Easy Omega-3 Smoothie: https://vitapurahealth.com/easy-omega-3-smoothie/.
- Omega-3 Smoothie: https://allnutribulletrecipes.com/omega-3-smoothie-recipe/.
- Omega Overture Mixed Berry Smoothie: https://www.driscolls.com/recipes/ omega-overture-mixed-berry-smoothie.

REFERENCES

1. No author(s) listed. 2008. Interim Summary of Conclusions and Dietary Recommendations on Total Fat & Fatty Acids from the Joint FAO/WHO Expert Consultation on Fats and Fatty Acids in Human Nutrition, 10–14 November, 2008, WHO, Geneva.
2. Agostoni C, Bresson J-L, Fairweather-Tait S, Flynn A, Golly I, Korhonen H, Lagiou P, Løvik M, Marchelli R, Martin A, Moseley B, Neuhäuser-Berthol M, Przyrembel H, Salminen S, Yolanda Sanz Y, Strain S (JJ), Strobel S, Tetens I, Tomé D, van Loveren H, and H Verhagen. 2012. Scientific opinion on the tolerable upper intake level of eicosapentaenoic acid (EPA), docosahexaenoic acid (DHA) and docosapentaenoic acid (DPA). EFSA Panel on Dietetic Products, Nutrition and Allergies (NDA). *European Food Safety Authority (EFSA) Journal*, Jul 27; 10(7): 2815. DOI: 10.2903/j.efsa.2012.2815.
3. No author(s) listed. 2010. US Department of Agriculture, US Department of Health and Human Services, Dietary Guidelines for American 2010; https://health.gov/sites/ default/files/2020-01/DietaryGuidelines2010.pdf; accessed 3/24/22.

4. No author(s) listed. 2005. The National Academies of Sciences, Engineering, Medicine. 2003 Dietary reference intakes for energy, carbohydrate, fiber, fat, fatty acids, cholesterol, Protein, and amino acids; https://www.nap.edu/catalog/10490/dietary-reference-intakes-for-energy-carbohydrate-fiber-fat-fatty-acids-cholesterol-protein-and-amino-acids; accessed 3/24/22.
5. https://www.mayoclinic.org/diseases-conditions/heart-disease/in-depth/omega-3/art-20045614; accessed 3/24/22.
6. https://www.webmd.com/heart/news/20090803/daily-omega-3s-recommended-heart; accessed 3/24/22.
7. Siscovick DS, Barringer TA, Fretts AM, Wu JHY, Lichtenstein AH, Costello RB, Kris-Etherton PM, Jacobson TA, Engler MB, Alger HM, Appel LJ, Mozaffarian D, and American Heart Association Nutrition Committee of the Council on Lifestyle and Cardiometabolic Health; Council on Epidemiology and Prevention; Council on Cardiovascular Disease in the Young; Council on Cardiovascular and Stroke Nursing; and Council on Clinical Cardiology. 2017. Omega-3 polyunsaturated fatty acid (fish oil) supplementation and the prevention of clinical cardiovascular disease: A science advisory from the American Heart Association. *Circulation*, Apr 11; 135(15): e867–e884. DOI: 10.1161/CIR.0000000000000482.
8. Rimm EB, Appel LJ, Chiuve SE, Djoussé L, Engler MB, Kris-Etherton PM, Mozaffarian D, Siscovick DS, Lichtenstein AH, and American Heart Association Nutrition Committee of the Council on Lifestyle and Cardiometabolic Health; Council on Epidemiology and Prevention; Council on Cardiovascular Disease in the Young; Council on Cardiovascular and Stroke Nursing; and Council on Clinical Cardiology. 2018. Seafood long-chain n-3 polyunsaturated fatty acids and cardiovascular disease: A science advisory from the American Heart Association. *Circulation*, Jul 3; 138(1): e35–e47. DOI: 10.1161/CIR.0000000000000574.
9. Skulas-Ray AC, Wilson PFW, Harris WS, Brinton EA, Kris-Etherton PM, Richter CK, Jacobson TA, Engler MB, Miller M, Robinson JG, Blum CB, Rodriguez-Leyva D, de Ferranti SD, Welty FK, and American Heart Association Council on Arteriosclerosis, Thrombosis and Vascular Biology; Council on Lifestyle and Cardiometabolic Health; Council on Cardiovascular Disease in the Young; Council on Cardiovascular and Stroke Nursing; and Council on Clinical Cardiology. 2019. Omega-3 fatty acids for the management of hypertriglyceridemia: A science advisory from the American Heart Association. *Circulation*, Sep 17; 140(12): e673–e691. DOI: 10.1161/CIR.0000000000000709.
10. Plourde M, and SC. Cunnane. 2007. Extremely limited synthesis of long chain polyunsaturates in adults: Implications for their dietary essentiality and use as supplements. *Applied Physiology, Nutrition and Metabolism*, 32: 619–634. DOI: 10.1139/H07-034.

Index

A

ABI, *see* Ankle-brachial index
Acetylcholine (ACh), 41, 42
Age-related macular degeneration (AMD), 89, 90
Agricultural Research Service (ARS), 30
Alcohol metabolism, 39
Alpha-linolenic acid (ALA), 45, 48, 50, 100, 103, 105–109, 117, 118, 159
American Academy of Ophthalmology (AAO), 89
American Heart Association (AHA), 3, 54–56, 160
American Journal of Clinical Nutrition (2004), 88
American Journal of Clinical Nutrition (2020), 152
American Journal of Clinical Nutrition (2008), 13
American Journal of Physiology. Heart and Circulatory Physiology (2018), 102
Aneurysm, 61
Ankle-brachial index (ABI), 81
    cuff placement, 80, 81
    definition, 79, 80
    and endothelial dysfunction, 82
    home-style test, 80
Annals of Gastroenterology (2016), 86
Annals of the New York Academy of Science, 90
Annals of the Rheumatic Diseases (2016), 83
Antioxidant diet, 63
Antioxidants, 17, 25, 30–35, 39, 43, 45, 49, 53, 63, 72, 77, 92, 100, 123, 151; *see also* Omega-3 essential fatty acids
    benefits of, 33
    beta carotene, 27
    endogenous antioxidants, 24, 28, 29
    exogenous antioxidants, 24, 28, 29
    flaxseed, 25
    food-borne antioxidants, 28
    with free radicals, 28
    high ORAC-unit foods, 31
    premature aging prevention, 30
Applied Physiology, Nutrition and Metabolism (2015), 44
Aquatic food web, 131
Archives in Cancer Research (2017), 102
Archives of Cardiovascular Diseases (2009), 80
Archives of Medical Research (2012), 84
Archives of Ophthalmology (2003), 90
Arteriosclerosis, Thrombosis and Vascular Biology (2018), 69
Atherosclerosis, 78
    flaxseed, 99
    omega-3 FAs, 67–68
    plaque formation, 67
    schematic of formation, 66
    thrombosis, 67
Atherosclerosis (2019), 67

B

Basic Cognitive Aptitude Tests (BCAT) scores, 91
Beta carotene, 27
Biological Trace Elements Research (2021), 153
Biomagnification, 141
BioMed Research International (2014), 78
"Blood levels of long-chain n–3 fatty acids and the risk of sudden death," 3
Blueberries, 33–36
Brain, Behavior and Immunity (2013), 18
British Journal of Nutrition (1993), 103
British Journal of Nutrition (2011), 134
British Journal of Nutrition (2012), 64

C

Canadian Journal of Cardiology (2010), 48
Cardiology in Review (2014), 78
Cardiovascular Diabetology (2018), 70
Cardiovascular diseases (CVD), 3, 8, 11, 12, 34, 35, 41–44, 51, 53–56, 62, 67, 82, 85, 127
    age-standardized rate of deaths, 25, 26
    Type 2 diabetes, 69–70
Cellular and Molecular Biology (2010), 64
Center for Food Safety of the Government of Hong Kong Special Administrative Region, 156
Centers for Disease Control and Prevention (CDC), 39
Central European Journal of Immunology (2015), 78
Cholesterol, 5, 39, 53, 62, 68, 70, 143, 144, 147, 149
    high-density lipoprotein (HDL), 6
    low-density lipoprotein (LDL), 6
    triglycerides, 6–7
    very-low-density lipoprotein (VLDL), 6, 7

CHRISTUS Health and Pharco Pharmaceuticals, 155
Chronic kidney disease (CKD), 78, 84–86
   flaxseed, 112
   omega-3 FAs, 86
Circulation (2010), 78
Circulation (2019), 12
Circulation (2020), 51
Circulation Research (2012), 66
CKD, *see* Chronic kidney disease
Clinical Nutrition (2014), 88
Clinical Nutrition Research (2015), 45
Clinical Rheumatology (2019), 111
Cochrane Database of Systematic Reviews (2008), 70
Cod liver oil, 144–145
Cognitive impairment in aging, 78, 90–92
Comprehensive Physiology (2013), 84
Coronary artery disease (CAD), 78
Coronary heart disease, 2, 3, 8–10, 14, 19, 52, 54, 106, 134, 145
Covid-19, 29, 41
   and selenium deficiency, 152–155
Current Diabetes Reviews (2018), 71
Current Nutrition Reports (2021), 153
Current Pharmaceutical Design (2016), 99
Current Topics in Nutraceutical Research (2007), 112
Cutaneous and Ocular Toxicology (2019), 87
CVD, *see* Cardiovascular diseases
Cyanogenic glycosides (CNGs), 102–104

D

Dementia, 62
Diabetes Care (2014), 70
Diabetes Self-Management recommendations, 79
Diatoms, 7
"Dietary flaxseed as a strategy for improving human health" (2019), 120
Dinoflagellates, 7
Dry eye disease (DED), 89

E

"The effect of flaxseed in breast cancer: a literature review," 119
Endogenous antioxidants, 24, 28
Endothelium, 67, 69
   anatomy, 40, 41
   damages to, 41, 43–44
   endothelial dysfunction, 43
Endothelium-derived relaxing factor (EDRF), 42
Estradiol, 4, 6
European Cardiology Review (2019), 78
European Heart Journal Supplements (2002), 79
European Journal of Clinical Nutrition (2009), 106
European Journal of Clinical Nutrition (2019), 110
Exogenous antioxidants, 24, 28

F

Fats
   "bad cholesterol," 5
   "good cholesterol," 5
   healthy fats (*see* Omega-3 fatty acids; Omega-6 fatty acids)
   low-fat diet, 4
   monounsaturated fats, 5, 6
   polyunsaturated fats, 5, 6
   saturated fats, 4–5
   vitamin D, 4
Fatty acids (FAs), definition, 1
Fish
   cod fish, 138
   contaminants, 140
   content and constituents, 135–137
   cooking fish, 139
   eels, 145–146
   fish oil, 143–145
   health benefits of, 139
   herring, 138
   high levels of mercury, 141–142
   home delivery, 140
   roe and caviar, 146
   sardines, 135, 136
   sea urchin, 147
   seaweed, 147
   in shellfish, 142–143
   tilapia, 139
Flaxseed, 25, 33–36, 49–51
   absorbability, 105
   alpha-linolenic acid (ALA), 45, 48, 50, 100, 103, 105–109, 117, 118
   Arthritis Foundation lists, 109
   for atherosclerosis, 99
   bioavailability, 105
   for cardiovascular risk factors, 110
   chronic kidney disease, 112
   chronic systemic inflammation, 109
   for coronary artery disease, 110
   cyanogenic glycosides (CNGs), 102–104
   in daily diet, 125–127
   dietary recommendations, 100
   disadvantages, 105, 127–128
   golden flaxseed *vs.* brown flaxseed, 123
   health benefits, 101, 103
   lupus nephritis, 111
   macronutrients, 123
   metabolic syndrome, 109–110

Index

micronutrients, 100
in obesity, 111
oil and capsules, 124, 125
organic *vs.* non-organic flaxseeds, 122
osteoarthritis, 111
phytoestrogens, 99
polycystic ovary syndrome, 112
prostate cancer, 111
recipe books, 127
Recommended Dietary Allowance (RDA), 101
rheumatoid arthritis, 111
safety, 103
secoisolariciresinol diglucoside (SDG), 99, 119
supplementation recommendations, 117–119
supplement dosages, 107, 109
Type 2 diabetes, 110–111
for ulcerative colitis, 110
whole/ground flaxseeds, 123–124
Food-borne antioxidants, 28
Food Chemistry (2009), 33
Food Frequency Questionnaire (FFQ), 134
Four-day diet records, 44
Free Radical Biology and Medicine (1993), 30
Free radicals, 16–17, 23–25, 28–32, 40, 69
Frontiers in Aging Neuroscience (2018), 78
Frontiers in Cardiovascular Medicine (2022), 67
Frontiers in Endocrinology (2020), 72
Frontiers in Nutrition (2018), 119
Functional foods, 100

G

Glaucoma, 78
    age-related macular degeneration (AMD), 89, 90
    arterial blood vessels endothelium, 87
    definition, 87
    dry eye disease (DED), 89
    macular degeneration, 89
    omega-3 FAs, 87–89
    primary open angle glaucoma (POAG), 87
    risk factor, 87
Golden flaxseed *vs.* brown flaxseed, 123

H

Healthy food patterns *vs.* unhealthy food patterns
    high-carbohydrate diet, 45–46
    high-fat diets, 44
    high-sodium diet, 44
Heart
    anatomy, 46, 47
    arterial vessel compliance
        flaxseed oil, 50–51
        schematic representation, 49, 50

atrial fibrillation, 48
chamber contractions, 48
congestive heart failure, 46
ejection fraction, 47, 49
endocardium, 47
heart failure, 49
hypertrophy, 46
nitric oxide levels, 48
omega-3 FAs, 49
    American Heart Association (2003) recommendations, 54–56
    aortic valve stenosis, 51
    coronary arteries protection, 52–53
pumping action, 48
Herring, 138
High-carbohydrate diet, 45–46
High-fat diets, 44
High-sodium diet, 44
Homarus americanus, 149
Hospital Pharmacy (2014), 148
Hot-rod mitochondria, 16
Human and Experimental Toxicology (2002), 29
Human Nutrition Research Center on Aging (1999), 31
Hunter-scrounger's diet, 2
Hydrogenation process, 6
Hypertension, 78
    ACh, 42
    antioxidant diet, 63
    complications, 61–62
    omega-3 FAs
        deficiency and consequences, 63
        fish consumption, 64
        Omega-3 Index (O3I), 64–65
    omega-6 FAs, 63
    plasma ORAC measures, 63
    prehypertension, 59
    primary hypertension, 59
    risk factors, 60–61
    secondary hypertension, 60
    stage 1 (moderate), 59
    stage 2 (severe), 59
    Standard American Diet (SAD), 62
    US Department of Agriculture (USDA) Dietary Guidelines for Americans, 62, 63
    Western Pattern Diet, 62
Hypertension Research (2010), 63

I

Inflamm-aging, 90–92
International Journal of Molecular Sciences (2020), 78
International Urology and Nephrology (2016), 112

Investigative Ophthalmology & Visual Science, 90
Irritable bowel syndrome (IBS), 86–87

J

Journal of Cardiology (2010), 43
Journal of Cardiovascular Pharmacology and Therapeutics (2019), 68
Journal of Clinical Epidemiology (1995), 83
Journal of Clinical Hypertension (2014), 44
Journal of Crohn's and Colitis (2014), 86
Journal of Diabetes Complications (1996), 71
Journal of Diabetes Complications (2017), 73
Journal of Dietary Supplements (2011), 110
Journal of Food Science and Technology (2019), 102, 103
Journal of Hypertension (2018), 64
Journal of Medical Case Reports, 2015, 34
Journal of Molecular and Cellular Cardiology, 49
Journal of Nutrition (2005), 107
Journal of Nutrition and Metabolism (2012), 120
Journal of the American College of Cardiology, 2017, 25
Journal of the American College of Nutrition, 63, 106
Journal of the American Medical Association (JAMA), 19, 82
Journal of the American Medical Association (JAMA)— *Ophthalmology* (2014), 72, 78, 87
Journal of the Federation of American Societies of Experimental Biology (FASEB) (2021), 68
Journal of the Medical Association of Thailand, 2012, 34
Journal of the National Cancer Institute, 4
Journal of Vascular Surgery (2003), 82
Journal of Vascular Surgery (2014), 82

K

Keshan syndrome, 153
Kidney International (1995), 111
Kippering, *see* Herring
Krill oil, 148

L

L-arginine, 42, 43, 104, 105, 107
Life Sciences, 48
Lupus nephritis, 111

M

Macular degeneration, 78
Malondialdehyde (MDA), 30
McDonald's type diet, 16

Mechanisms of Ageing and Development (2014), 35
Medical Hypotheses (2020), 155
Mediterranean Diet, 3, 4, 12, 14, 43, 134
Mediterranean Diet Score (MDS), 135
Mercury, 141–142
Metabolic syndrome, 62, 109–110
Mollusks, 2, 142, 148, 151, 155
Monounsaturated fats, 5, 6
"My Plate" app, 161

N

Nature Communications (2021), 11
Neurology (2012), 91
Neurotransmitters, 42, 45, 48
New England Journal of Medicine (NEJM), 39, 42
Nitric oxide (NO), 42
Non-steroidal anti-inflammatory drugs (NSAIDs), 84
Nori, 147
Nutrients (2020), 89
Nutrients (2021), 44, 134
Nutrition and Dietetics (2019), 82
Nutrition Research (2017), 64
NutritionData, 161

O

Obesity/overweight, 62, 83, 111
Office of Dietary Supplements Health Professional Fact Sheet, 160
Okinawa
    diet, 35, 36
    lifespan, 25–27
Omega-3 essential fatty acids (FAs), 9, 49, 160
    in adults and seniors, 120
    anti-inflammatory and endothelial protective effects, 10
    atherosclerosis, 67–68
    beneficial effects, 45
    benefits of, 25
    breakfast recipes
        blueberry omega-3 breakfast bowl, 163–164
        greek muffin-tin omelets with feta and peppers, 165–166
        hearty oatmeal pancakes with flax and chia seeds, 162–163
        homemade açaí bowl, 164
        Mediterranean tofu scramble, 166
        mini blueberry muffin recipe, 164–165
    cardioprotective effects, 10
    in chronic kidney disease, 84–86
    coronary heart disease, 2
    crickets, 8
    deficiency, 2, 119

Index

dinner recipes
  baked Mediterranean fish recipe, 172
  green tea poached salmon with ginger lime sauce, 171–172
  harvest squash medley, 174–175
  salmon salad with parsley and capers, 173
  simply poached salmon, 173
  slow-roasted salmon with fennel, citrus and chiles, 174
eicosanoids, 11, 120
in fish, 3, 4
  cod fish, 138
  contaminants, 140
  content and constituents, 135–137
  cooking fish, 139
  eels, 145–146
  fish oil, 143–145
  health benefits of, 139
  herring, 138
  high levels of mercury, 141–142
  home delivery, 140
  roe and caviar, 146
  sardines, 135, 136
  sea urchin, 147
  seaweed, 147
  in shellfish, 142–143
  tilapia, 139
grubs, 8
heart
  American Heart Association (2003) recommendations, 54–56
  aortic valve stenosis, 51
  coronary arteries protection, 52–53
hypertension
  deficiency and consequences, 63
  fish consumption, 64
  Omega-3 Index (O3I), 64–65
jellyfish, 155
lunch recipes
  grilled sauerkraut avocado sandwich, 170–171
  Mediterranean shrimp quinoa bowls recipe, 167
  Mexican sardine salad stuffed avocados, 167–168
  salmon cakes with creamy ginger-sesame sauce, 168–169
  spinach salad with winter squash and walnuts, 170
  tuna and green bean salad, 169–170
Mediterranean diet, 134
mollusks, 2
mussels and abalone, 155
octopus, 150–151
Omega-3 Index, 2, 8–9, 13–16, 121–122
osteoarthritis (OA), 83
oysters and clams, 151

peripheral artery disease (PAD), 82–83
peripheral neuropathy, 71–72
phytoplankton, 7
plant oils, 9
premature aging prevention, 18
pro-inflammatory agents, 10
retinopathy, 72–73
rheumatoid arthritis, 84
scallops, 151–152
seal oil, 132
shellfish allergy, 148–149
shrimps and prawns, 147–148
squid, 150–151
Type 2 diabetes, 69–73
vegetable sources, 133
Western diet, 134
Omega-3 Index (O3I), 2, 8–9, 83, 121–122, 134, 160
  and blood pressure, 64–65
  in different countries, 14, 15
  risk zones, 13
Omega-6 fatty acids, 2, 7, 8, 161
  eicosanoids, 11, 120
  in foods, 121
  healthy ratio, 12
  pro-inflammatory agents, 10
  recommendations, 121
  types, 11
  Western diet, 4, 9, 11, 12
ORAC, *see* Oxygen radical absorbance capacity
Organic *vs.* non-organic flaxseeds, 122
Osteoarthritis, 83–84
  flaxseed, 111
Oxygen free radical, 16
Oxygen radical absorbance capacity (ORAC)
  antioxidant analysis, 31
  antioxidant capacity for selected foods, 31, 32
  blueberries *vs.* flaxseed, 33–36
  definition, 30
  high ORAC-unit foods, 31
  laboratory method, 30
  slow aging, 31
  USDA Database, 33

P

Paleolithic diet, 1, 8
Pathogens (2014), 86
Patient Preference and Adherence (2016), 70
Peripheral artery disease (PAD), 78, 79
  omega-3 fatty acid deficiency, 82–83
Peripheral neuropathy, 71–72
Pharmacognosy Review (2010), 32
Phytonutrients, 31
Phytoplankton, 131–133
PLoS One (2015), 70
Polycystic ovary syndrome, 112

Polyunsaturated fats, 5, 6, 103, 104
Poultry Science (2000), 100
Preventive Medicine, 2004, 9
Primary open angle glaucoma (POAG), 87
Progress in Lipid Research (2016), 14
Prostaglandins, Leukotrienes and Essential Fatty Acids (2006), 87

Q

Quicksilver, *see* Mercury

R

Reactive Oxygen Species (ROS), 17, 23, 24, 28–31, 39–46, 48, 60, 67, 69, 72
Resveratrol, 29
Rheumatoid arthritis, 83–84
Rheumatology (2020), 83

S

Sardines, 135, 136
Saturated fats, 4–5
Science Daily (2015), 71
Science Daily (May 14, 2018), 48
Scientific Reports (2020), 65
Selenium deficiency, 152–155
Sepsis, 30–31
Shellfish allergy, 148–149
Six-day meal plan
    breakfast recipes
        blueberry omega-3 breakfast bowl, 163–164
        greek muffin-tin omelets with feta and peppers, 165–166
        hearty oatmeal pancakes with flax and chia seeds, 162–163
        homemade açaí bowl, 164
        Mediterranean tofu scramble, 166
        mini blueberry muffin recipe, 164–165
    desert and smoothie recipes, 175
    dinner recipes
        baked Mediterranean fish recipe, 172
        green tea poached salmon with ginger lime sauce, 171–172
        harvest squash medley, 174–175
        salmon salad with parsley and capers, 173
        simply poached salmon, 173
        slow-roasted salmon with fennel, citrus and chiles, 174
    EPA + DHA content, 159
    food charts, 159
    lunch recipes
        grilled sauerkraut avocado sandwich, 170–171
        Mediterranean shrimp quinoa bowls recipe, 167
        Mexican sardine salad stuffed avocados, 167–168
        salmon cakes with creamy ginger-sesame sauce, 168–169
        spinach salad with winter squash and walnuts, 170
        tuna and green bean salad, 169–170
    Mayo Clinic recommendations, 159–160
    omega-3-rich recipes, 162
    plant sources of, 160–161
    recommended dietary allowance (RDA), 159
Spain, Mediterranean diet, 3, 4
Standard American Diet (SAD), 12, 62; *see also* Western Pattern Diet
SuperTracker tool, 161

T

T2D, *see* Type 2 diabetes
TBARS, 30, 31
Telomeres, 17, 18
Therapeutic Advances in Ophthalmology (2019), 87
Tilapia, 139
Translational Vision Science and Technology (2018), 88
Triglycerides, 1, 6–7
Trolox, 30, 33
Type 2 diabetes (T2D), 41, 43, 45, 62, 63, 77, 78
    cardiovascular disorders, 69–70
    fish intake, 70–71
    flaxseed, 110–111
    heart and blood vessel disease, 71
    peripheral neuropathy, 71–72
    retinopathy, 72–73
    signs and symptoms, 69
    wound-healing, 73

U

Ubiquinol, 17
US Department of Agriculture (USDA) Dietary Guidelines for Americans, 62, 63

V

VIAGRA®, 42
Vitamin A, 31
Vitamin D, 4
Vitamin deficiency, 1

W

Walnut-crust ginger salmon, 34
Well balanced diet, 12
Western Pattern Diet, 4, 9, 11, 12, 44, 62, 134
World Journal of Gastroenterology (2016), 86